FATAL SEQUENCE

Kevin J. Tracey

FATAL SEQUENCE

THE KILLER WITHIN

DANA
PRESS NEW YORK • WASHINGTON, D.C.

D
DANA
PRESS

The Dana Foundation
745 Fifth Avenue, Suite 900
New York, New York 10151

Dana Press
900 15th Street, NW
Washington, DC 20005

DANA is a federally registered trademark.

ISBN: 1-932594-06-X

LIBRARY OF CONGRESS CATALOGING-IN-PUBLICATION DATA
Tracey, Kevin J.
    Fatal sequence : the killer within / Kevin J. Tracey.
        p. cm.
    ISBN 1-932594-06-X (hardcover)
    1. Septicemia in children—Patients—Biography.
    2. Burns and scalds in children—Patients—Biography,
    I. Title.
    RJ320.S45T73 2005
    617.1'1'0083092—dc22
                                    2004025330

Design by Kachergis Book Design
Printed by Edwards Brothers Incorporated

To J.F., the real Janice

Contents

FATAL SEQUENCE

Introduction

TUESDAY, MAY 28, 1985. It was a birthday party for a one-year-old, but the cake had no candle. Oxygen was in use nearby, and Fire Department rules prohibited open flames. The birthday girl was Janice, a patient on the burn unit of New York Hospital. Silver foil balloons twitched gently against the ceiling, proclaiming ONE YEAR OLD in blue and green pastel letters. A circulating fan on the wall moved the humid air gently as doctors, nurses, and family passed around pieces of cake. White bandages covered Janice's arms, legs, and torso, an intravenous bottle hung from a pole, and a green-screened cardiac monitor beeped beside her crib. The guests laughed as Janice smeared chocolate frosting across her white bandages and onto the rails of her crib. Mercifully, the burn had spared her sweet face, and Janice's bright blue eyes sparkled.

This was more than a celebration of Janice's first year of life, because no one had really expected her to last this long. One month earlier she had been scalded by boiling water spilled from a spaghetti pot. The baby had crawled between her grandmother's legs just as she had turned from the stove to drain the pasta water. The woman stumbled and never made it to the sink. Boiling water had poured onto Janice, burning more than 75 percent of her body. Now the people who had kept her alive were rejoicing in her survival. After weeks of long days filled with round-the-clock care, the burn unit staff had grown to love the innocent and persistently cheerful child. It had not all been for nothing. Janice was going to make it after all.

Janice's four weeks in the burn unit had been an unimaginable nightmare for her parents. Terrifying dreams would also haunt Janice's doctors and nurses for years. She had been to the operating room for major surgery to excise the burned areas, which were then covered with skin grafts. She had lived through daily dressing changes that lasted more than an hour each, and she had been on and off a respirator three times. She had received gallons of intravenous fluids and tube feedings, and six different antibiotics. Somehow she had made it this far, battling through one complication after another caused by her scalding. Her wounds had left her widely exposed to the harshness of the surrounding microbial world. Antibiotics, ointments, and dressing changes did not stop the microbial invasion—germs had entered her bloodstream, and her organs had shut down. Her immune system fought back—launching a vicious attack—but as in an urban battle in streets crowded with people, where killing is indiscriminate, the immune attack had not only killed invading bacteria but severely damaged her organs as well. Janice's lungs, kidneys, liver, and heart were damaged by what is known as severe sepsis.

Severe sepsis is a modern-day pestilence, a leading cause of death worldwide. In the United States alone it kills 215,000 annually, making it the third leading cause of death, after cardiovascular disease and cancer. More people die every day from severe sepsis (589 deaths a day) than from acute heart attack. The medical cost of its treatment in the United States exceeds $17 billion annually. Severe sepsis can occur, as in Janice's case, after a burn injury, but it develops more commonly in other kinds of patients. Typical conditions that predispose patients to develop severe sepsis include cancer, multiple traumas from a motor vehicle accident, and pneumonia or other infections. Severe sepsis can even develop spontaneously in previously healthy patients, especially those at the extremes of life—the very young and the elderly.

I was one of Janice's doctors in the burn unit 20 years ago, and I was frustrated by the lack of answers to fundamental questions about severe sepsis. What is it, really? How does it happen? Why do some people get it but not others? What does it feel like? And how does it kill? Consumed by the need to know what had happened to her, and hoping to find new treatments, I began a career in scientific research shortly after I treated her. Janice's story compelled me to study sepsis. Since that time researchers have learned that severe sepsis occurs when patients' own molecules turn against them; they suffer and die at the hands of their own immune systems. They are wounded when molecular weapons launched against microbes damage the body's own tissues and organs. Severe sepsis is a failure of the weapons-control system. During a routine infection or injury, your immune system responds to protect you, but it is a controlled response in which the release of weapons is held in check. Just enough are fired to effectively protect you from microbes. In a patient with severe sepsis, however, this carefully orchestrated response spins wildly out of control, instigating a sequence that can kill the patient as well as the microbes.

In a surprising twist to this story, my colleagues and I recently discovered that the brain is a master command-and-control center for the immune system's weapons. Messages to the immune-microbial battlefield are carried by nerves that deliver critical orders from the brain, keeping the attack on track, restraining its magnitude, and preventing it from veering off to damage bystander organs. The brain exerts a powerful constraint on the immune response, preventing it from becoming too activated. Your brain can protect you against lethal complications from commonplace infections, cuts, scrapes, and minor injuries, such as a urinary tract infection or a pimple. Neural pathways lying deep within the brain can also prevent the severe sepsis sequence.

Janice's story encompasses not only the 25 days that she spent in the burn unit. It also describes her scientific legacy, the work of countless scientific investigators who are unraveling the mysteries that obscured severe sepsis at the time she was hurt. Janice's real identity remains confidential. I did not review her records to write this book; it is not a journalistic account. Instead, these are my recollections of her struggle to survive her dual assaults: from the scalding and, afterward, from her own immune system. All the medical events described here are true. I did not make recordings or take notes during Janice's hospitalization, so the conversations recounted here are reconstructed from my memory. The dialogue and specific daily activities here are composites, re-created from discussions and clinical events and distilled from the thousands of patients I have treated. Many, like Janice, suffered combined blows from their own immune systems and doctors' ignorance. In preparing this book I interviewed sepsis survivors, clinicians, and scientific investigators; their quotations are exact, as noted. Other names have been changed to protect confidentiality.

Today a new class of drugs can block the immune system's molecular weapons, significantly improving the quality of life for hundreds of thousands of patients. The scientific path that led to this major advance did not follow a straight line but took a more erratic course, marked by sharp turns, accidents, and surprises. It is not possible here (or perhaps in any single text) to list all the investigators who worked on these problems, or to describe their individual contributions to the research that led to new treatments. Instead, I have chosen to highlight a few specific discoveries in order to give a glimpse into the way basic laboratory research, far from the patient's bedside, can occasionally identify new approaches to understanding the complexity of the immune system and suggest new methods to control it. Only a small fraction of scientific experiments actually "work." Most of the time the results are equivocal; sometimes they are even confusing. Pivotal experiments move understanding forward, on a track that everyone hopes will circle back to the patient's bedside as a future therapy and, perhaps, a cure.

one

The ER

FRIDAY, MAY 3, 1985, 5:35 P.M. Janice, 11 months old, was playing on the kitchen floor in her grandmother's walk-up apartment in a Brooklyn brownstone. It was hot in the kitchen because Cecilia was cooking pasta in a ten-quart pot that bubbled furiously on the stove. Janice's parents were due home from work, and Cecilia wanted to have the spaghetti on the table when her daughter and son-in-law walked through the door. The steam from the pot fogged the room. Janice was busy playing with her teddy bear, giggling and screeching as she crawled across the black-and-white-checkered linoleum floor. She stopped right behind her grandmother, between the kitchen sink and the stove.

Cecilia tasted a strand of pasta, pronounced it done, snatched the heavy pot of boiling pasta from the stove top, and turned toward the colander waiting in the sink. Then she stumbled on Janice, spilling the pot's 212-degree contents onto her only grandchild. Hearing screams, a neighbor ran into the kitchen. Cecilia had carried the hysterical child to the kitchen table and was struggling frantically and clumsily to remove Janice's steaming-hot clothes. The neighbor and Cecilia undressed Janice, a task hampered by the intense heat of the clothes, which burned the fingers of both women. After stripping Janice down to her onesie and diaper, they called 911.

5:45 P.M. The New York City Fire Department ambulance arrived with two emergency medical technicians. The EMTs entered the third-floor apartment to find Janice crying, gasping for air between choking sobs. Cecilia was standing in the center of the living room, cradling the scalded child, now wrapped in a clean baby blanket. The EMTs gently pried Janice loose from her trembling grandmother's protective embrace, the kind of desperate hug that tries to shield the innocent. They buckled Janice onto the stretcher with wide black Velcro belts across her knees and chest, carried her down the stairs, and loaded her into the back of the ambulance.

The ambulance was crowded, crammed with fifteen thousand dollars' worth of essential equipment. Packed into the 45 square feet in the back of the "bus" were green oxygen tanks bracketed to the wall, a portable respirator, a battery-operated cardiac defibrillator and monitor, intravenous catheters, blood pressure cuffs, a pneumatic antishock suit, fire extinguishers, and dozens of boxes of assorted bandages, gauze, and medications. Effective emergency medical "pre-hospital" care is critically dependent on properly evaluating the injury, assessing the victim's status, and preventing or minimizing the development of further damage. The highly trained EMTs knew that a major problem facing a young burn victim is severe dehydration. Large scald injuries in children can cause tremendous fluid losses that in turn can cause blood pressure to plummet suddenly, even to lethal levels.

The EMTs clamped Janice's stretcher to the floor of the bus, attached a black Velcro blood pressure cuff to her right biceps, and measured her blood pressure. They recorded it, along with her heart rate and respiratory rate, on a flow sheet attached to a weathered clipboard. Parked curbside in the sun, the ambulance was uncomfortably hot. The two EMTs began their struggle to insert an intravenous catheter into Janice's left arm. She screamed inconsolably as they splinted her elbow and applied a temporary tourniquet to bring up the antecubital vein. The tiny, deep blue vein appeared near the surface of the skin at the bend of her arm, and while one EMT held Janice's splinted arm fast against the stretcher, rigidly tight and still so that the needle would not cut clear through the vein, the other slid the catheter over the needle, into the vein. They connected the catheter to the intravenous line and began to infuse "Ringer's lactate," a sterile saltwater solution, to prevent dehydration. They wrapped the IV site in dry gauze because tape would not adhere to the wet burns.

The medics battled to stabilize Janice, in a stressful scene that could have been lifted straight from a war movie. Tears trickled down her unburned face, wetting her blond hair, which hung in streaks across her face and ears. The EMTs injected some codeine to take the edge off her pain and prepared to depart for the hospital. One stayed in the back to monitor Janice; the other climbed behind the wheel. He radioed Janice's medical information to the emergency room at New York Hospital. The ER cleared a room in preparation for Janice's arrival, and the triage nurse called the burn unit: "Eleven-month-old female with whole-body scald injury; ETA, 20 minutes."

The driver switched on the lights and siren and turned the ignition key to start the diesel engine. Lights flashing and siren wailing, the ambulance pulled into the traffic and headed toward Seventieth Street and York Avenue, in Manhattan. The EMT riding with Janice continued to check her blood pressure and other vital signs every five minutes, a process that would be continued by countless doctors and nurses, around the clock, for the next four weeks. The claustrophobic space smelled of diesel exhaust, and the noise of the siren was deafening. As the ambulance sped along the Interborough Parkway, about halfway to the hospital, Janice suddenly stopped breathing. Her face turned deep blue, and then her heart rate began to slow. The EMT placed an oxygen mask over her mouth and nose, but her heart slowed further, and then it stopped.

The ambulance was bumping and rocking back and forth as the EMT tried to gather together an endotracheal tube, a plastic tube to be inserted in Janice's windpipe, and a laryngoscope, a handheld instrument used to hold the mouth open and pull the tongue forward during insertion of the tube.[1] He knew that Janice would die unless he immediately inserted the tube into her airway, but the bus was moving and shaking so much that he kept bouncing out of his seat and falling across Janice. Inserting an endotracheal tube into a small child is a very difficult task even under optimal conditions. The EMT realized he couldn't do it in these circumstances. With all the shaking and jumping, there was a good chance that he would stick the tube into Janice's esophagus instead of her trachea, an error that could kill her. By now her heart had been stopped for two full minutes—time had nearly run out. He yelled for the driver to stop, and the bus screeched onto the shoulder of the highway in a cloud of dust and gravel.

The rocking, seasick movement stopped, but before the EMT had even tried to insert the endotracheal tube, Janice's heart miraculously came back to life, and she started breathing again. Within seconds, it was as if nothing at all had happened: Janice was crying, breathing, pink, and had a strong pulse and heart rate. The EMT was drenched in sweat from the heat and the stress of knowing that Janice had essentially died and come back, and that while he had been responsible for her, he had been helpless to alter the course of events. Worse, he knew that she could crash again and that if she did, she would probably not come back a second time. He yelled "Let's go!" to the driver, who accelerated the ambulance back into the traffic lane.

Unfortunately, the driver, who had been watching the events unfold in the back while the ambulance was parked, was "task-saturated" and misjudged the speed of the traffic coming up behind him. The ambulance's lights were flashing and its siren was blaring, but as the driver pulled back onto the highway, the ambulance was struck from behind by a car speeding up the right-hand lane. The collision caused the ambulance to swerve back into the breakdown lane and travel 200 feet before again swerving, this time back into the traffic lane. The impact had crushed the ambulance's rear bumper and damaged the front end of the colliding car. Janice was still completely unstable, and the driver did not know if her heart would keep going. It was a fender bender, but he could see that the other driver was not hurt, and there was no time to stop and exchange insurance information, so he floored the accelerator and continued full speed to the hospital. His patient's life was hanging in the balance, and he figured that he could exchange paperwork with the other driver in the parking lot at the ER, if they ever got there.

Janice was now the critically ill passenger of a vehicle chauffeured by a participant in a motor vehicle accident who had left the scene of the accident. The driver of the other car followed the ambulance closely all the way, pounding the horn, and screaming obscenities out the window, demanding that the ambulance stop. After a 15-minute ride that seemed far longer, both vehicles finally pulled into the ER parking lot. The irate driver jumped out of his car, still yelling and cursing at the ambulance driver, who was by now assisting the other EMT in unloading the crying Janice. A burly security guard approached the driver, hushing him. Once the EMT from the back of the bus had delivered Janice to the relative safety of the emergency ward and was back in familiar hospital surroundings with his colleagues and other people who could take over, he began to shake and sob quietly, overcome by the void that set in as his stress ended.

Janice's ambulance driver knew well the route and all the shortcuts to New York Hospital because in his eight-year EMT career he had delivered many other scalded children to this burn unit. Severe scald injury is a leading cause of pediatric trauma in the United States. One hundred thousand children are scalded annually by spilled food and beverages severely enough to require hospitalization. Usually this happens when a toddler pulls a container of hot liquid or food off a countertop or, as in Janice's case, bumps into an adult carrying hot beverages or food. Children from 9 to 21 months (like Janice) are at the highest risk of scald injury.

Injuries like Janice's are avoidable. The American Burn Association has developed a well-researched list of specific recommendations that can help to prevent scald injury in children. Every kitchen should have a designated "safe area," where children can play out of the traffic path between the stove and sink. High chairs and play areas must be located at a safe distance from stove tops, hot liquids, and other cooking hazards. Whenever children are in the kitchen, cooking should be done on the back burners of the stove, with pot handles always turned away from the front of the stove. Appliance cords and towels should be coiled and placed away from counter edges. Hot items should be placed in the center of the table on nonslip place mats rather than a tablecloth to prevent children from inadvertently dousing themselves by pulling on the overhanging edges of the tablecloth. Adults carrying children should not simultaneously carry hot liquids. Hundreds of childhood scald injuries like Janice's occur when an adult is jostled or stumbles, spilling hot liquid onto the child. Children should never be allowed to remove food from a microwave oven without adult supervision. Microwave ovens produce pressurized steam that when released will quickly burn exposed skin on the face, arms, and hands. Heated food should be removed from the microwave by an adult, cautiously, after a delay of one or two minutes from the end of the cooking cycle and only when there are no children underfoot. (More detailed recommendations can be found at www.ameriburn.org.)

6:30 P.M. I met Janice in the emergency room, less than one hour after she had been scalded. It was my second year as a doctor, and I was training to become a surgeon. Four years of medical school, a busy internship in surgery, and countless hours in operating rooms and emergency wards had familiarized me with the sights of cancer, gunshot wounds, head injuries, and ravaged human frames twisted and contorted by injury and infection. But I was completely unprepared for the sight of a little strawberry-blond child lying under the bright lights on the shiny chrome table. Underneath her pink teddy-bear-festooned blanket, Janice was covered in blistered and shredding skin. The boiling water had converted her back, arms, and legs into a coagulum of dysfunctional tissue. Using bandage scissors, the nurses and I cut off Janice's pink onesie and disposable diaper to reveal the evidence of thermal destruction. Thin, delicate, pristine skin should have enveloped her, not this blistered, oozing, disfigured mess. Her back, scalp, arms, legs, and neck were covered with welts and blisters that seemed to grow as I watched.

A burn is damage to the skin caused by heated liquids, flames, hot objects, chemicals, or electricity. The skin is one of the body's major organs, with a mass accounting for between 15 and 20 percent of body weight. It is composed of 60 percent water and 40 percent solid material. The solid materials in skin are made of proteins and lipids (fats) that have been incorporated into skin cells. Each cell is a viable life-form that can grow and propagate itself. Skin cells live in a surrounding matrix that is both strong and flexible, like a scaffold that holds the cells in organized compartments. At normal body temperatures, the protein and fat molecules are vibrant and mobile, jiggling and humming in place like guitar strings. This molecular movement is the atomic dance of life that imbues cells with the ability to metabolize fuel, regenerate, and perform their specialized functions.

The outer layer of the skin, visible on your own body surface, is the epidermis, a thin coating of (mostly) dead cells and other detritus that protects the layer of cells lying just underneath. The epidermis is continuously replaced by growing cells that reproduce and move upward and outward to the surface. Popular commercially available exfoliating skin-care products are abrasives that remove the outermost layer of dead tissue and detritus from the epidermis. Heat or friction applied to pressure points on the skin—for instance, from that infrequent tennis match or autumnal Saturday morning bout of raking leaves—causes blisters by pulling the epidermis loose from the tissues beneath.

Underneath the epidermis lies the dermis, a thicker layer of tissue that varies significantly in size and shape over various body parts and among individuals. A number of specialized cells also reside within the dermis, including hair follicles, sweat glands, and cells called melanocytes, which produce melanin, a pigmented molecule that colors the skin. Exposure to sunlight causes tanning because melanin absorbs ultraviolet light, becoming darker. The dermis also houses cells that provide the front line of defense against infection and invasion by germs. Called Langerhans cells, these cellular infantries are scattered throughout the skin in a weblike pattern that forms a network critically positioned to confront any microscopic invader or germ. Langerhans cells even gobble up nonviable material, such as ink squirted into the dermis from a tattooist's needle. After ingesting ink granules and packaging them into intracellular vacuoles, the Langerhans cells enter a hibernation-like state and cease moving forever. This serves the tattooist's purpose well because the individual grains of tattoo ink inside the Langerhans cells remain in one place rather than floating around in the extracellular matrix. Thus, even though the dermal scaffolding is replaced, the tattooist's ink grains are safe and still, immobilized inside the cells.

The extracellular matrix of the dermis is held together by bands of stretchable protein fibers, composed primarily of collagen, that surround the cells, the hair follicles, the sweat glands, and the sebaceous, or oil-secreting, glands. Healthy dermis is sustained by a rich blood supply, which delivers oxygen and nutrients through small arteries and carries away carbon dioxide and other cellular waste in the veins for delivery to such toxin-processing organs as the lungs, kidneys, and liver. The dermis also contains nerve fibers that sense pain; when activated by heat or pressure they signal the brain, which instigates an appropriate protective response (for example, withdraw from heat).

Sensory input from the skin is constantly fed into the brain, but most of these signals are ignored unless there is a crisis. For instance, as you sit reading this book with your legs resting on the ottoman, you are largely unaware of any sensation of pressure on the backs of your calves. But when you turn your conscious attention to them, you can immediately become "aware" of the sensory information provided by the nerves in your skin. A severe or painful stimulus, like a burn wound, registers in your consciousness immediately, and without any action on your part. A burn injury activates the pain fibers to transmit deep, paralyzing signals that your brain processes into sensations of local pain, nausea, fatigue, weakness, stress, and fear.

The depth of a burn wound is related to the temperature of the burning substance and the exposure time. Superficial burns, or first-degree burns, are generally minor and heal in three to five days with little or no specific medical therapy. They look pink or red, are painful to the touch, and are dry without blisters. Partial-thickness, or second-degree, burns are more serious because the damage extends deeper, into the underlying dermis. They are colored bright pink or red and are blistered, moist, wet, and weeping. They are extremely painful and begin to swell almost immediately. Skin grafts are not usually required, because the dermis can heal, but this may take up to three weeks, and sometimes skin graft surgery is performed to hasten recovery.

The most serious burns are the full-thickness, or third-degree, burns, which destroy both layers of the skin. The damage may extend to the underlying fat, muscle, and bone. These burns are dry, leathery wounds that can be bright red, waxy white, or charred brown, and clotted blue veins can often be seen coursing through the burned area. They are less painful than the more superficial burns because the nerves to the affected area have been destroyed; the victim may not even be able to feel the examiner touching the injury. Skin grafting is required for effective healing. Boiling water (at 212 degrees Fahrenheit) causes a third-degree burn in under one second of exposure time; even relatively cooler hot water, at 155 degrees Fahrenheit, causes a third-degree burn in under two seconds.

6:45 P.M. Janice was agitated and moaning despite the codeine she had received. I suppressed thoughts about the pain caused by Janice's partial-thickness burns. Like other medical professionals, I had learned to block out the suffering of the innocent. We must, really, in order simply to perform our jobs. We *will* feel the pain at some future time, probably as a dream in the middle of the night that will replay the horrible ER scene in slow motion—a repetitive, sleep-interrupting show, unedited so as to elicit all the emotion, tears, anguish, and suffering that the brain had blocked during the actual live performance. In the ER that night, my brain edited the material in real time. It excised most of the emotional content, sterilized the scene, and deleted Janice's pain from my reality. This unfettered me; my less cluttered brain could then focus on the overlapping checklists of essential items. It was as if some deeper brain region was saying to me, "Concentrate on Janice's medical needs, not her pain; her survival desperately requires your undivided attention, right now, not your tears."

I examined Janice carefully, searching for evidence of other injuries or broken bones. She was well nourished, her face retained the puffy pink cheeks of her infancy, and her thighs and arms were layered with little bundles of baby fat. I wrote my clinical findings in her chart, including a sketch of her body and the location of her burns. Doctors record objective, stereotypical phrases in these situations, such as "previously healthy 11-month-old female" and "burns covering the back and extremities," without ever adding what they really feel. They would never describe the sweet, unburned face of a child who could be their own—so small, innocent, and afraid. Using a reference card depicting the percentage of total body surface represented by each major body region for an 11-month-old girl, I calculated that 75 percent of her skin surface had been severely injured with second- and third-degree burns. A simple formula based on her age and the percentage of burns placed Janice's odds for surviving at about 25 percent.

Third-degree-burned skin is no longer "skin" but a lifeless, coagulated protein mess known as eschar. Eschar is like a growth medium for germs, which multiply at astounding rates in the tender nutrients provided by cooked flesh. Instead of flexible molecules that jiggle and hum with vibrancy and life, the proteins composing eschar have been converted by heat into rigid, sticky, lifeless clots, like an egg white on a hot frying pan. Before heating, the egg white is fluid, clear, and capable of supporting and nourishing life-forms as complex as a growing chick. But heat "denatures" the egg white, destroys molecular structure, and renders it biologically useless to a developing chick. In the open air a cooked egg white is, however, a fantastic culture medium that can nourish much simpler life-forms, like bacteria. See for yourself, if you dare. Simply leave a cooked egg white in a warm place for a few days, then observe and smell the evidence of new life breeding on the denatured proteins. Germs will breed wildly on the lifeless tissue, and as they grow and expand, they will devour and decompose the denatured protein into a putrefied, smelly mass. Lying there in the ER, covered in eschar, Janice was intimately enveloped in a grotesque blanket of denatured proteins. And unseen bacteria had already begun moving into their newfound dwelling place.

Destruction of skin renders burn victims defenseless against invasion by bacteria. Microorganisms dominate all life on this planet, covering everything with a fine veil of bacterial life, a "microbiological skin." Every detail, from the grandest mountain peak to the tiniest hair on a bumblebee's leg, is enshrouded in microscopic life. Janice was now easy prey for these germs. They could replicate in the nutritious eschar without any harassment from the local immune system in her skin, because it had been killed by the heat. There was no way for the immune system to send in replacements either, because the blood vessels to the area were sealed shut by the scalding. Janice was exquisitely vulnerable to an infection that could kill her in the next few weeks. Boiling water had destroyed her skin, and with it her front-line defensive barrier against microorganisms.

By the time Janice arrived at the ER, bacteria in the air, on her teddy bear blanket, on her grandmother, the neighbor, and the EMTs had already begun to establish themselves on Janice's eschar. In the ER, even doctors' neckties carried pathogens from room to room, and patient to patient. In the course of a typical day, bacteria frequently gain access to your tissues and bloodstream. Germs enter your body every time you cut yourself shaving, scratch a mosquito bite, or get a paper cut. In the overwhelming majority of these cases, the germs do not take hold, because millions of years of vertebrate evolution have endowed you and other humans with an elaborate and powerful immune system that provides a nearly perfect defense against germ attack. In the 11 months preceding her scald injury, Janice had never developed any serious infections or major health problems. Her relatively young immune system had successfully defended her from a daily onslaught of infectious opportunities. Countless times her skin had defeated an overwhelming bacterial force, a veritable surrounding army of attacking germs too numerous to count. Until the day she was burned, she had repelled the microbes without ill effect, and she had thrived. But now the burn injury had wiped out large parts of Janice's defensive front lines, enabling microbes to begin growing in Janice's eschar. They were already there, replicating and propagating. It was as if they were biding their time, fortifying their positions in preparation for their territorial expansion into her bloodstream and internal organs.

Normal, healthy skin forms a strong physical barrier between the germs in the outside world and the critical internal organs. Skin supports and maintains defensive cells poised to attack bacteria at the first signs of invasion. Langerhans cells are "macrophages," members of the extended white blood cell family, which also includes neutrophils, monocytes, lymphocytes, mast cells, and dendritic cells. White blood cells are born in the bone marrow and released into the bloodstream, from where they are dispatched to various destinations, such as the spleen, the liver, and the lymph nodes. These sites are the bastions and strongholds of the immune system. Macrophages take up residence in the skin, lungs, and other sites of potential attack, where they lie in wait, ready to devour invading bacteria. They sit beneath the radar of your consciousness, all the while surveying their landscape for a probing germ or invader to enter through small breaches in the skin.

Macrophages, like all cells, are endowed with their own microscopically thin "skin," as it were, composed of a fatty cell-surface membrane. The membrane is decorated with proteins that extend outward like the tentacles on a jellyfish. These proteins serve as docking stations, among other roles, where molecules approaching the macrophage are captured. Called receptors, these docking stations are exquisitely sensitive to molecules produced by invading microorganisms. Like the sensory nerve endings in your skin, which can detect pain, pressure, and temperature and relay this information to your brain for processing and to evoke an appropriate response, the receptors on the macrophage surface provide a means for the macrophage to sense the goings-on in its environment. For example, specific individual molecules from a bacterium can fit into a receptor like a key into a lock, an event that notifies the macrophage that a microbial invader has slipped into the fold. This process provides the macrophage with information about the nature and intensity of the attack or threat, and the identity of the bacterium.

The receptor is like a string crossing through the macrophage's skin. One end of the string lies outside the cell, and the other dangles on the inside. When a molecule docks outside the macrophage, the part of the receptor that protrudes inside the cell changes shape. Like the child's game of telephone, in which a string pulled tightly between two aluminum cans transmits sound as a vibration along the line, the changing shape of the receptor inside the macrophage is the signal that there are foreigners outside. The surface of a macrophage is covered with thousands of receptors, each of which can interact with only one, or at most a few, specific molecules. Some receptors bind hormones, others bind factors produced by the immune system, and still others bind toxins produced by microbes. Individual cells rely on this system as a basic communications network. Cells can respond to molecules produced by nearby cells, or to molecules arriving from a great distance, carried through the bloodstream, or along a nerve. A specific molecule interacts with a specific receptor to elicit a stereotypical response in the cell. When bacterial molecules bind to the macrophage's skin, as if banging at the gates, the defending cell is incited to furious activity.

The presence of microbes whips the cells of the immune system into a frenzy, converting them into angry, biting, and weapons-firing machines that focus all their molecular resources on killing the bacteria. The immune system cells are extremely good at this task; they identify the bacteria as foreign invaders and kill them. No salve, no antibiotic solution, and no sterilizing cream even comes close in defensive effectiveness to the army of immune cells lying in your skin, on the ready and at your disposal. You may not be conscious of your dependence on these dermal cellular protectors, but they are there, keeping the germs out of your bloodstream and preventing infection. Your very survival is dependent on your macrophages' ability to effectively engage the microbes and stymie their advance. The defensive lines hold because evolution has endowed the fighters with powerful molecular weaponry that kills microbes before they can establish a foothold, cause an infection, or spread through the bloodstream.

The encounter between bacteria and macrophages in the battle zone causes the macrophages to become "activated," an offensive posture that directs a lethal molecular barrage. Information about the nature of the attacker is shuttled rapidly from protein to protein inside the macrophage, arriving ultimately in the macrophage's nucleus, the cell's command-and-control center. There, genes are switched on and off in response to an alarm that something bad has happened at the cell surface. The activation of these genes is like the orders a platoon sergeant barks to his troops: "Bacteria present. Attack. Fire at will."

Weapons produced and released by the macrophages do a first-rate job of killing bacteria, and make the dermis a downright hostile environment for germs. Some of these molecular weapons are proteins that drill holes into bacterial cell walls, which explode because the bacteria themselves are pressurized like balloons. An eclectic collection of specialized cells join the macrophages in the fracas. Neutrophils are especially good at making lethal, ozonelike molecules and hypochlorous acid, the active ingredient in laundry bleach. Lymphocytes make antibodies that stick to the bacteria, surrounding their surfaces and targeting them for destruction by macrophages and neutrophils.

During the battle against the microbes, the immune system's cells are in constant communication with each other by means of the production and release of molecules known as cytokines, a family of proteins that interact with specific receptors on immune cells, as well as such cells as neurons, muscle cells, and the endothelial cells lining blood vessels. Cytokines with names like TNF, HMGB1, IL-1, and interferon-γ modulate the troop activity, direct the movement of the fighting cells, and coordinate the battle attack positions. When a cytokine arrives at its destination, it binds or docks to a receptor on a cell in the area, causing that cell to change its activities and behavior in a specific manner. In this way cytokines control important functional changes in individual cells, coordinating the behavior and goings-on of diverse cells in a complicated immune response.

Cytokines produced by macrophages, neutrophils, lymphocytes, and other immune cells can serve as a call for reinforcements, because they exert a powerful attraction on white blood cells, which will crawl through a blood vessel wall to enter the battle when ordered to do so by cytokines. Cytokines released at the site of infection may travel to the nearby skeletal muscle cells, directing the release of amino acids as needed to fuel the immune cells in battle. Cytokines can interact with endothelial cells in blood vessels, causing them to become sticky or to dilate, effects which can either slow or increase blood flow to the battle as necessary to either increase or decrease the number of fresh white blood cell troops. Cytokines are key to the effectiveness of a coordinated immune attack.

During a low-level or minuscule invasion, as occurs perhaps when you prick yourself with a pin, or scratch your gums with dental floss, the resultant antimicrobial cellular battles are relatively quiet and localized. Few germs are involved in these situations; the macrophages usually kill them quickly and prevent their spread without your notice. The immune response in these trivial cases may seem rather innocuous, but it is critical to prevent bacterial growth and infection. If these early and limited defensive steps fail, and the bacteria develop a firmer foothold and replicate, then a heavier immune response will be initiated against the bacteria now entrenched in infected tissue. Large numbers of white blood cells with the intimidating name polymorphonuclear leukocytes arrive via the bloodstream, firing their toxic weapons into the bacterial maelstrom.

It is likely that you will feel pain from this pitched, contaminated battle and become conscious of the local proceedings. Collateral damage begins to occur, and just as noncombatant bystanders can be killed in their own homes during an urban battle, so too can normal host cells be killed by macrophage-derived toxins. Your skin at the site may liquefy as a painful boil develops. Bacteria grow in this fluid, producing larger amounts of toxins, which elicit an even larger immune response. The side effects of this battle and the now locally widespread use of molecular weapons kill not only the bacteria but some of your own normal skin cells as well. The boil will grow, creating painful pressure on the surrounding tissues, which by now are crammed full of white blood cells and bacteria. At the center of the tenderness—the part that makes you wince when you bump it inadvertently—your own skin cells have died. They were killed in the battle between your immune system and the bacteria. The molecular weapons of the immune cells and cytokines, and the effluent from the skin cells dying in the boil, stimulate the pain fibers in your skin. Your brain receives these electrical signals, deciphers the message entrained in their frequency and distribution, and you feel the pain.

The overwhelming majority of fights between the immune system and microbes pass unnoticed by you; the immune system inevitably wins the day, stopping bacterial advances in their tracks without causing signs or symptoms. Evolution molded these immune responses into a highly effective defense that restricts bacteria to the skin and other body surfaces where they are first encountered. The immune system's cytokines were not meant to spill into the bloodstream, though; this is a dangerous scenario.

In 1974, Lewis Thomas, the great immunologist and writer,

presaged what we have since come to understand is the consequence of an excessive, systemic release of cytokines from the immune system. In *The Lives of a Cell* he wrote: "Our arsenals for fighting off bacteria are so powerful, and involve so many different defense mechanisms, that we are in more danger from them than from the invaders. We live in the midst of explosive devices; we are mined . . . we are likely to turn on every defense at our disposal; we will bomb, defoliate, blockade, seal off, and destroy all the tissues in the area . . . It is a shambles." Unfortunately, that is exactly what can occur, for instance, in cases of a perforated appendix or colon. Cytokines are produced in massive amounts, saturating the tissues around the infected bowel and then spreading via the bloodstream to distant organs. These cytokines, so effective when activated in a controlled local environment, are deadly if they spread into the bloodstream.

Once cytokines enter the circulation they can cause fever, aversion to food, and potentially lethal damage to the heart, kidneys, and lungs. The immune system's powerful weapons, amazingly effective when aimed directly at the invaders in a local environment, can kill normal cells too. Armed, dangerous, and uncontrolled, cytokines are quickly distributed by flowing blood, killing indiscriminately and nonspecifically. We did not know any of this at the time of Janice's hospitalization, but the damage caused by the immune system's cytokine response to infection can kill even previously healthy young individuals like Janice.

7:15 P.M. In the ER, I drew a diagram in Janice's chart, showing the sites of her wounds and noting the severity of the scald damage. Partial-thickness burns, whose damage is limited to the more superficial layer of the skin, will usually heal without surgery. Cells in the underlying dermis will eventually proliferate and form a scar to cover the burned epidermis. Full-thickness burns, however, require surgery for timely healing. Damage to the deepest layers of the skin not only kills the cells necessary for healing, but it also destroys the small blood vessels traversing the dermis and carrying needed vital oxygen and nutrients. Unfortunately, most of Janice's wounds were full thickness. The boiling hot water had soaked into her clothes, trapping the heat against her skin, prolonging the exposure time, and causing deeper burns. Full thickness burns are shiny, white, and toughened because the epidermis, hair follicles, and pores become coagulated in place. Where there should have been a gentle pinkness from light reflected off the tiny red blood vessels perfusing her dermis, there lay instead large patches of pale white, gruesome-looking eschar. Within 15 minutes of meeting Janice, I had completed my estimation of her probable long-term needs for extensive surgery (100 percent); her probable chance of developing a severe infection (more than 95 percent); and, as previously noted, her probable chance of going home alive (no better than 25 percent).

There were other pressing requirements that we had to consider in the early care of Janice, as with other injured or burned patients. We had to exclude the possibility that she had sustained other soft-tissue injuries or broken bones, which might have occurred if she had also been struck on the head or torso by either the dropped spaghetti pot or her falling grandmother. Donning sterile yellow gloves, I gently palpated Janice's arms, legs, ribs, and skull, feeling along the smooth bony surfaces for any irregularities that would have indicated a fracture. I looked into her mouth and upper airway, probing with a wooden "tongue stick," to find any evidence that she might have inhaled the scalding water or burned her throat and lungs. Every five minutes the nurses measured her blood pressure, calling out the numbers with a regular cadence before recording them on her chart.

Glass bottles hung from a pole, dripping Ringer's lactate into her veins to counteract the dehydrating effects of her burn injuries. Ringer's lactate, a sterile solution that contains salts, lactate, glucose, and water, is a standard intravenous fluid used to supply volume and electrolytes to patients who are either dehydrated or unable to consume fluids so as to prevent them from becoming dehydrated. The intravenous catheter placed by the EMTs was still functional, but it had a narrow bore (22 gauge) that would provide significant resistance to flow; it would not do, because we would not be able to infuse her intravenous fluids fast enough. Janice needed larger catheters, and I would have to put them in soon. I gently pressed on her abdomen, checking for any localized tenderness or masses caused by bleeding from a ruptured organ, artery, or vein. She cried through the entire exam, and she needed intravenous morphine to obtain even minimal relief. It was time to move her upstairs to the burn unit.

two

The Burn Unit

The burn unit of New York Hospital was on the seventh floor of the Payson Pavilion. Two- and four-bedded patient rooms lined both sides of a long central hallway that emptied into a spacious glass solarium facing south, overlooking the East River and the tree-filled, parklike campus of Rockefeller University. During a recent major reconstruction, the burn unit was moved to a new building, and the original Payson 7 Burn Unit was converted into a modern office suite for the Department of Surgery. Now the center corridor of the old burn unit is lined with file cabinets, and a drop ceiling hangs low over office cubicles on both sides. The rooms that once housed the patients now enclose doctors' offices with desks displaying photographs of smiling families. But the renovation has not erased the old burn unit; those who knew it, past patients and caregivers, can still feel its presence on the seventh floor. Listen carefully as you walk through the offices, and you too might hear the ghostly sounds of heels clicking down the long gray linoleum floor, now covered by new carpeting. The burn unit Janice and I knew is preserved forever behind the Sheetrock, the acoustic tiles,

28

and the faces of the smiling children peering out from the picture frames arranged on the desks of the secretaries and doctors.

FRIDAY, MAY 3, 1985, 7:30 P.M. The ER nurse and I exited the elevator on the seventh floor, crossed the main hallway that ran the length of the hospital, pushed Janice's stretcher through the swinging door, and entered the burn unit. A single window, crisscrossed with reinforcing wire, was positioned at eye level in that door, but I never saw anyone gazing through it, either in or out. This window was not installed for gawking; its only discernible purpose was to embellish the burn unit gateway, the sole route of entrance and egress. Perhaps in the course of its long existence this window had prevented a collision or two between folks simultaneously rushing the door from both sides, but I doubted it. Fast-moving traffic was not a major problem here. Once a patient entered through this door, it was a long time before he or she departed. Janice, the newest and youngest burn victim, rolled into the unit.

Rooms on either side of the hallway housed the burn victims. The "nearly recovered" occupied the rooms closest to the door. Most of these "long-termers" had lived in the unit for two or three months. Their discharge dates were approaching, and they could often be found talking to each other near the wire-windowed door, leaning on the door frames of their rooms, or chatting on their black bedside telephones, inevitably streaking the handsets with telltale gobs of white antibiotic cream from their wounded faces and hands. Each day the medical team discussed the patients and their progress, deciding whether any patient in the deeper rooms, at the other end of the hallway, was healthy enough to move closer to the swinging door, to the recovery end. Patients, doctors, and nurses all tracked the patients' movement as they inched toward the exit, like a horse race running in slow motion. The lucky ones progressed a step, or a room, closer to home, an event that always elicited smiles, congratulations, and general celebration.

As you walked deeper into the burn unit, the severity of the burn wounds increased. An imaginary line separated the healing and mostly well patients from the critically ill and newly burned. Old-timers did not cross the line or mingle down here; they already had served their time and did not return voluntarily. Levity and banter, which punctuated the conversation nearer the door, disappeared here. The rooms at the far end of the hallway were individual intensive care units, each stocked with the most advanced monitoring equipment available at the time. The game was different down here: patients struggled to survive one day at time, as their families milled about in the hallway, praying and asking questions, always imploring with their eyes, occasionally verbalizing the tough questions to the staff.

Halfway down the hallway, on the left, was the nursing station, a landmark housing a clerk's desk and two long, low gray Formica counters. These served triple duty as charting stations for doctors and nurses, telephone booths, and staging areas for incoming supplies, charts, and order books. The clerk, donning a navy blue hospital uniform jacket with her name stenciled in white cursive across the left breast pocket, sat at her desk facing anyone passing in the hallway. She was the gatekeeper, positioned on the threshold dividing the burn unit into the standard hospital rooms to one side and the intensive-care-unit rooms to the other. The gatekeeper's head shook ever so slightly as we pushed Janice past. She did not minister directly to these patients, but they were all her patients just the same.

During the upcoming weeks the clerk would spend countless hours processing Janice's paperwork, her doctors' orders, and hundreds of slips requesting blood tests, X-rays, specialty physician consults, and pharmacy orders. Several times every day she would speak with Janice's parents and her grandmother, Cecilia. On their way in and out of Janice's room, the family would stop by the desk to chat; the clerk would come to know them intimately. A bond would form between them, one stronger than they could have imagined, forged by the stress of what would happen to Janice. This personal and intense closeness would not develop with the doctors, nurses, or any other hospital employees, just the clerk. Janice's parents would confide in her alone, revealing their darkest fears, spilling out the whole tragic story. It was the gatekeeper who would learn the most about their anguish, shame, and pain.

The clerk would watch their tears fall, cry with them, and note sadly the progressive changes in their physical state: weight loss; dark, shadowy circles spreading under gloomy eyes; and depressed countenances that would scar their faces with creases. Soon it would be impossible to see the evidence that Janice had inherited her ready smile from these faces.

The clerk knew well the grave dangers hovering in the rooms past her halfway point, where intensive care lasted for days or weeks at a time, and patients lapsed in and out of consciousness, largely unaware of their surroundings. She had seen too many freshly burned patients roll past her desk on the way to their rooms, only to leave weeks later, this time covered by a sheet, passing her desk on the way to the morgue.

The critically ill patients were attended to by medical staff attired in disposable clothing: light blue paper masks, floppy mesh hats, oversize white paper booties, and yellow cloth-paper gowns. The outfits made everyone look like they belonged to the cast of a cheap science fiction movie about strange germs from outer space invading Earth. The disposable clothes were essential to the concerted and continuous effort to reduce the likelihood that bacteria carried along on clothing would be brought into contact with the burn victims. Everyone entering Janice's room was required to change into these outfits. Families and visitors bunched up in small groups just outside the doorways, fitting themselves in paper-wear stacked on the stainless steel carts lining the hallway. The ubiquitous yellow outfits were sentinels, reminding us that the bacteria were everywhere, always ready to infect the burn wounds, threatening life. Conversational tones were subdued and guarded, spoken like quiet prayers, summoning hope in the hearts of the lemon paper-covered people.

In the event of a large-scale disaster or emergency, nearly all of the rooms on both ends of the burn unit could be converted into intensive care rooms. Usually, however, all the critically injured patients were housed in the rooms past the nursing station. Recovery from these intensive care unit beds was never certain, and it occurred only after a struggle. Time was marked from the burn injury itself, a sort of tragic time zero denoting exactly when life was forever altered. For the lucky ones, progress and milestones after time zero were celebrated: the first day off the respirator, the first day sitting up in a chair for a meal, the first day to speak. The loving families watched these events unfold like small miracles in this burn unit, with tender emotions as indelibly recorded in their memories as those of the first birthday cake, or first step. Whenever a patient showed signs of improving, the optimism was palpable. It was not discussed, but the staff needed these signs of progress in order to keep going, to keep the whole process from seeming like an endless, frustrating, losing battle. Each recovery of function was celebrated as a joyous second beginning, even when it might have seemed a trivial repeat of a previous first, like eating solid food again for the "first" time. Progress was precious on Payson 7.

Most critically ill patients in the intensive care unit cannot think or speak clearly. They lie silent, disoriented, confused, unresponsive, or comatose. Perhaps it is a blessing that new memories are not formed; painful experiences are not registered or stored in their brains. The events of their intensive care unit experience will be largely inaccessible to their future mind's eye, never to appear uninvited to disturb the bliss of some future picnic or family reunion. Survivors may well be haunted by daydreams and nightmares of their actual burn injury, but with rare exceptions they recount only vaguely, as if through a dense fog, their intensive care unit experience. Vague recollections of the ICU are not unique to burn patients; survivors of major surgery or other injury recount similar sensations of being disconnected from their environment. Maybe it is their brain's way of protecting them from developing permanent psychological scars.

For the families, however, it is a different story. Relatives and friends remember it all. Their memories are not impaired, and they recall clearly every painful ordeal, every day of suffering, every needle stick, every surgery, every delayed discharge date, every setback, and every new infection. Even years later they will recall with vivid clarity moments when they received bad news, describing in frightening detail the entire scene: the doctor's or nurse's name, the look on her face, and that they were standing next to the fresh daisies in the pale blue vase on the bedside table.

The doctors and nurses of the burn unit sometimes remember the tiniest details, too. There was the 55-year-old man who was transferred to the unit from upstate New York after the plane he was piloting through a thunderstorm crashed on its final approach to a local airport. I admitted him to the burn unit at 2 a.m., more than eight hours after the crash. He was burned over 90 percent of his body, but he was alert, fully conscious, lucid, and talkative. Scared and anxious, he clearly wanted to give me as much vital information as he possibly could, including family contact information, his past medical and surgical history, and the list of his daily medications.

The dimly lit room reeked of jet fuel and burned skin. He talked a lot, recounting the precise details of the crash and explaining that at the last possible moment he had managed to raise the nose of the plane sharply up toward the soft tops of tall pine trees rather than smashing directly into the thicker tree trunks at a steeper angle of decline. This skillful maneuver had probably saved the lives of his three passengers, who had walked away from the crash site, not needing hospitalization. Unfortunately, the pilot had been trapped in the wreckage when the spilled jet fuel ignited.

Firefighters had extinguished the flames, extracted him from the crumpled cockpit using the Jaws of Life, and airlifted him to the burn unit. Now he was lying on his back, his entire body covered in bulky white dressings, his lungs damaged from smoke inhalation, but talking incessantly, as if he believed that as long as he was talking there was a slim chance that he would survive. He described his business career, detailing the hurdles he had overcome in order to build his company's manufacturing operation to the point that it now employed 350 people in his small upstate New York hometown. He talked virtually nonstop for two hours, until his lungs began to collect fluid and he became short of breath.

Even then he struggled on, the stories coming more slowly as his speech became labored. His respiration worsened, eventually becoming so inefficient that we had to insert an endotracheal tube and connect him to a respirator. The breathing tube, wedged between his vocal cords, finally silenced him. Thus quieted, he mutely developed severe sepsis. His subsequent course was complicated by worsening lung damage, shock, kidney failure, and, after seven days, brain death. Had he survived, I know he would not have remembered our long, mostly one-sided chat, and, mercifully, he would have recalled neither his terror nor his pain. Depressed brain function, confusion, and altered levels of consciousness inevitably occur when the immune system's weapons reach the bloodstream, damaging all the organs, including the brain.

7:45 P.M. Also fully alert, a crying, sobbing Janice was admitted into the intensive care end of the burn unit, in the second room on the left past the nursing station. It was a four-bedded room, but for now she was its only occupant. Her crib had been set catty-corner under a window on the far side of the room. It was properly called a crib, but to me this intensive care unit version had always looked more like a cross between a steel shipping crate and a tiger cage. Rather than the gentle, fluid curves and soft white colors one normally associates with a baby's crib, Janice's "crib" was a squared-off, silver-painted, steel-framed rectangle made of vertical rails, like a prison cell that someone had turned into a crib by removing the top. A cardiac monitor with a green screen displaying a yellow electrocardiograph tracing hung at eye level from the wall just adjacent to her crib, beeping in rhythm with her heart.

The sides of the crib could be lowered to provide complete access to the patient, and this we now did in preparation for inserting intravenous and intra-arterial catheters into her leg. The intravenous line was necessary to deliver the relatively large amounts of fluid Janice would need to prevent dehydration. It also provided access to her veins for injecting pain medications and antibiotics. The arterial catheter served two other vital functions: it was connected to a monitoring device that displayed her blood pressure, and it was a source for her blood, a sort of hematological spigot that could be opened periodically to provide samples. Twice a day a small amount of her blood was siphoned off and sent for measures of oxygen, carbon dioxide, and blood sugar (glucose) and other tests.

We had to insert these catheters into Janice's femoral artery and vein, because the skin overlying the other major vessels in her body was burned. The femoral vessels, protected by her diaper, had not been burned, and they were large enough to accept relatively big catheters. The needle insertion point to hit these vessels lies where the top of the thigh meets the abdomen, in the sensitive groin area. This location was not usually chosen for this purpose, because the catheters would be in place for a long while. Every time Janice moved her legs, the catheters would move a little bit as well. Movements of the catheters where they penetrated the skin could widen the insertion holes or dislodge the catheters completely, scenarios that significantly increased the risk that the lines would become infected from the bacteria in her groin. But we had no other choice locations in which to place these catheters. The alternative sites in her arms, neck, and chest had all been burned.

I injected lidocaine into her groin, and Janice began to cry. The unburned and previously quiet pain nerves in the region were firing signals to her central nervous system, notifying the deepest regions of her brain that something was clearly wrong in the area of her femoral vessels. The technology for injecting needles and placing catheters in children has thankfully improved in the last 20 years. Now topical anesthetic creams and salves are universally available to effectively eliminate the pain of needle sticks. We did not have such methods at that time, however, and Janice cried, hard. An orderly from the emergency room arrived just then to reclaim the stretcher we had used to move Janice. "Mike" the orderly had an 8-month-old daughter of his own at home who had kept him up most of the night before, crying because of a middle ear infection. Now the sound of Janice crying transfixed him in the doorway. He stood there for several minutes, growing ashen-faced, glancing from Janice to me and the nurse, and back again. Then he shook his head once, murmured something I could not hear, and sullenly pushed the stretcher out of the room.

Just hours earlier, Janice had been playing on the floor in her steamy hot kitchen, oblivious to everything but her grandmother and teddy bear. Now her world was a steel cage in the burn unit. Of course the nurses and I didn't discuss it—the stark contrast between her previously safe, peaceful, and happy life and the present. Everything had turned on her, instantly transforming her familiar home routines into a strange, solemn, terrifying new reality. We focused instead on placing the catheters, working silently. A few minutes later the anesthetizing effects of the lidocaine mercifully dulled the pain fibers, and Janice stopped crying. I passed a long plastic catheter through a needle into her femoral vein; backed out the steel needle, leaving an 18-gauge plastic tube inside her vein; and then sandwiched the needle in a plastic housing that I stitched to her skin.

A glass bottle of Ringer's lactate hung from a stainless steel pole at the head of her crib, and the liquid now flowed freely into her femoral vein. The nurses placed a Foley catheter into her urinary bladder and measured the volume of urine that filled the tiny bag. Fluid in and fluid out: these would be monitored every hour for the rest of Janice's hospitalization. Urine production is a sign of kidney function that can reflect the hydration status of the injured patient. Severely burned children are extremely sensitive to dehydration because the burn wound itself allows massive evaporative fluid loss. Before the technology for intravenous needles and sterile solutions had been invented, patients with major burn injury used to die from dehydration, sometimes within a few hours of the burn.

Janice's blood pressure, heart rate, respiratory rate, and fluid balances, as well as her laboratory results and other data, were recorded on flow sheets. When fully unfolded, the flow sheet for a single day was nearly three feet long. By the end of each full day, both sides would be covered with the details of her treatment, medications, and nursing notes. These data and notes would be recorded, one sheet for each day, for the next four weeks. Stretched end-to-end for her entire hospitalization, the flow sheets would eventually run 25 yards, a repository of clinical information that memorialized Janice's progress and setbacks from the time she entered the emergency room. The staff studied these sheets, searching for patterns, clues, and trends indicating that Janice was getting better, or worse. Had she gotten enough intravenous fluid? Made enough urine? Was that a new trend in her blood pressure and heart rate? Was enough oxygen getting to her organs? And what about that white blood cell count? A vigilant watch was kept for any early signs of infection, an hourly survey for any indication that an infection was developing. Some of the signs were more important than others, especially those that can develop even before fever comes, such as a fall in platelet count, a rise in white blood cell count or glucose levels, or a change in mental status.

8:15 P.M. I performed a neurological exam on Janice, noting that she was alert and awake, moving all of her extremities voluntarily and in response to specific stimulation. Her pupils were 3 mm across, constricted normally to light, and her extraocular movements were not limited. She was crying, her facial muscles were symmetrical, and her tongue was in the midline. Her reflexes were symmetrical and normally reactive for her age. On these relatively crude tests of brain function, Janice received a passing grade.

These exams were our window into Janice's brain, a simple method to observe whether her brain's command-and-control functions were intact. For young children these tests and "coma scales" assign scores for eye opening, vocalization, and motor activity. The highest scores are given for spontaneous eye opening, cooing and babbling sounds, and spontaneous movements. The lowest scores are given for absence of eye opening even in response to pain, moaning or no verbal response, and abnormal movements associated with deep neurological damage. Janice started her new life in the intensive care unit with high test scores, indicating that her nervous system was continuing to function. For now, it was still running her physiological show.

11 P.M. Janice had been "resuscitated" with intravenous fluids and was continuing to receive enough fluids to prevent dehydration.[2] Her wounds were covered in Silvadene cream, a dense white ointment impregnated with the antibiotic silver sulfadiazine. Silvadene reduces, but does not eliminate, the risks of severe sepsis hanging over seriously burned patients like a sword of Damocles. The smelly white goo kills some of the microbes that live and reproduce on burn wounds. It has an acrid, too-sweet odor like a rotten pumpkin, that seems to settle at the back of your throat, lingering there whenever you are on the burn unit. Years later the smell of Silvadene still takes me back to that distressing place. The Silvadene-smeared burns were covered in fluffy white dressings that darkened in streaks as the ointment seeped through the gauze and oxidized, staining the wrappings a dirty brown and black.

It was time to insert the nasogastric tube, a four-foot-long plastic hose the thickness of a straw that is used to either pump out the stomach or pump in tube feedings. I threaded the tube through Janice's left nostril and advanced it down the back of her throat, pushing gently until it reached her stomach. The nurse taped the protruding part to her forehead, carefully securing it so that it would not be pulled out—either as a deliberate act by Janice, or accidentally by the staff. She connected the tube to a pump that would deliver a liquid formula at a rate calculated to sustain Janice's metabolism and nutritional status. For the next few weeks Janice would lose all interest in food and drink as a result of the combined effects of her burns, her pain, and the immune system's weaponry circulating in her blood. This lack of appetite would make it impossible to feed her with baby bottles.

This problem was compounded by the fact that Janice, like most critically injured patients, would soon develop a high metabolic rate that, unless balanced by nutritional intake, would rapidly deplete her vital stores of calories, protein, and fat. Like an engine in a parked car running with a wide-open throttle, Janice's metabolism would begin racing, and unless she received enough fuel to maintain it, she would starve to death. We knew that her metabolic rate would more than double within 48 to 72 hours, meaning that she would need to consume at least two times more calories than normal simply to prevent starvation. She was at risk of burning up her precious internal fuel supplies and losing weight while lying still in bed.

To understand Janice's metabolic responses to injury, consider that your body produces and utilizes energy to maintain the chemistry of life and to produce work (for example, exercise). Weight gain occurs when caloric intake exceeds calories lost to metabolism and work. Weight loss occurs when metabolism and work use more calories than have been consumed. Body weight is regulated within a narrow range, around an individual set point. The set point controls body weight by altering metabolism; body weight and metabolic rate tend to change in opposite directions. For instance, when an obese individual is placed on a reduced caloric intake, there is a corresponding decrease in metabolic rate that defends against weight loss, preserves body mass, and causes hunger. The brain works overtime to maintain body weight at a relatively high set point. The obese subject may be overweight, but the brain's response to caloric deprivation is similar to a thin person's. In both cases the set point triggers a coordinated response that says, in essence, GO GET FOOD. It works the other way too, because force-feeding thin volunteers significantly increases their metabolic rate, so that immediately after cessation of force feeding, the subjects burn off the extra fat and return to their previously normal body weight.

The controlling center of this set point resides deep in the brain. Known as the hypothalamus, it functions like a thermostat to precisely regulate metabolic rate and body weight. Normal adults typically experience some weight gain with aging; an average 25-year-old can expect to gain approximately 25 pounds over 40 years. But this is a relatively small amount of weight gain when compared with the amount of food consumed during this time period—that same individual will have consumed more than 18 tons of food.

You might expect that Janice's metabolism would slow down after her injury, so that her body could protect itself against the depletion of her internal fuel stores during her incapacitation. Indeed, that is exactly what happens to noninjured, healthy subjects; fasting or starvation causes the metabolic rate to slow to the absolute minimum rate needed for vital organ function. During food shortages, our early ancestors would lie low in their caves or dens, and their decreased metabolic rates would prolong the life span of their internal fuel reserves until they could eventually find food. This picture changes, however, if a major trauma or infection is superimposed on the fasting state.

During the early period after a major injury, the metabolic rate does indeed slow down, but this energy-sparing metabolic response lasts only 24 to 72 hours. Within three or four days a massive surge in metabolism occurs, driven by increasing levels of the stress hormones epinephrine, norepinephrine, and cortisol. This hormonal "stress response" increases the metabolic rate in cells. The hormone surge causes metabolism to race despite the absence of energy intake. In the short term this stress response is extremely beneficial to the injury victim. It facilitates rapid access to fuel in order to support wound healing, and it provides the fuel required to meet the demands of the immune system as it produces cytokines and wages an incessant war against the microbes. The speeding metabolism is part of the "fight or flight" response that can lead to feats of extraordinary strength in times of battle, on the athletic field, or at the scene of a motor vehicle accident.

After the acute threat is resolved, and the fight-or-flight mechanisms switch off, the host feels drained and exhausted, like the stricken EMT who delivered Janice to the ER. Nature never intended, and evolution did not select for, the prolonged increase in metabolism that can occur in today's ICUs. The fight-or-flight response evolved as a way to survive a sudden threat with a burst of energy that would last just long enough for the individual to resolve the confrontation and run back to its burrow. Janice lay in a modern intensive care unit that could keep her and other critically ill and injured victims resuscitated and sustained with intravenous fluids and respirators, in a state of protracted fight or flight that might last for weeks, or even months.

Janice would be sustained with a liquid diet pumped through her nasogastric tube in quantities sufficient to meet her increased metabolic needs. This approach can prolong life and bypass evolutionary pressure. Our ancestors did not survive comparably severe injuries and infection; they were simply eliminated from the gene pool. During this phase of increased metabolism, injured patients actively degrade their own vital body proteins, dissolving their own muscles and tissues and sending them into their urine. It is as if modern medical care and advanced ICU support systems have unveiled the "normal" metabolism of the dying. Mother Nature requires the terminal animal to degrade its own proteins and excrete nitrogen prior to becoming a carcass. In dying we become legumes! How parsimonious.

Your brain normally controls calorie consumption and food intake by regulating appetite. A "feeding center" is situated in the lateral hypothalamus, and a "saticty center" in the medial hypothalamus, near the bottom of your brain, behind your eye sockets. When nerves in the satiety center become activated, they inhibit the feeding center, causing loss of appetite. Stimulation of nerves in the feeding center significantly increases appetite and results in behavioral changes that increase food intake. Animals develop an aversion to food and weight loss if the feeding center is destroyed or inhibited. Since Janice's hospitalization, we have learned that cytokines are among the most powerful appetite suppressants; they both suppress the feeding center and stimulate the hormones that increase metabolism after injury or during critical illness.

Janice was not hungry, because her hormonal, metabolic, and cytokine responses to injury inhibited her feeding centers. She lacked any desire for food. To prevent her from starving and burning up her own precious stores of fat and protein, we fed her a concentrated liquid diet. A square blue pump hanging on the steel pole next to her crib pumped the high-protein, high-fat, high-calorie dietary formula directly into her stomach through the feeding tube. Twenty-four hours a day, whether her brain was hungry or not, Janice would receive enough calories to meet her basic metabolic needs. The milky white diet was the fuel she would need to fight, and hopefully heal, her wounds, and to mobilize her immune system to protect her from infection.

From the time she arrived on the burn unit, Janice was always under the watchful eye of a nurse. The Payson 7 nurses all received specialized training in burns and intensive care; many had also received training in pediatrics and postsurgical nursing care. They were dedicated specialists who watched Janice at all times, checked her vital signs every 10 or 15 minutes, and monitored all aspects of her treatment. She slept fitfully in her bandages, awakening every 10 to 15 minutes with a whimper and sob.

Before her burn injury, Janice would occasionally wake up at 2 or 3 a.m., falling back to sleep only after her mother had held her close in the rocking chair and given her a warm bottle of milk. Mealtimes with her family were the "main event" for Janice, marked by peals of laughter around a crowded table. She played with her food, made faces, and turned her nose up in protest at some spoonfuls. Then she would suddenly open her mouth wide and, looking like a baby bird, wait for her cereal and baby fruit to be deposited into her gullet. A camera was always near, ready to capture Janice's newly developing repertoire of facial expressions, some shy and others silly. Janice ate in her high chair, perched like a princess, ruling all that she surveyed simply by raising an eyebrow, pointing a finger, or chirping those special sounds unique to 11-month-old children.

I remember the pictures of Janice playing with her food, wiping applesauce across her face, forehead, and hair, and sweeping her crackers from her tray and onto the floor with a smile. Color pictures of her family at dinnertime were carefully arranged on the wall of the burn unit above the crib where she lay sedated, swathed in bulky dressings over her arms, legs, back, and chest. Now she received nutrition from a machine that pumped formula through the tube in her nose. This little Janice was so unlike the one in the picture; how could she be the same?

One picture showed Janice cradled in her mother's arms, drifting to sleep while sucking on a bottle in her nursery at home, peacefully smiling into the eyes of the woman who had delivered her into the world. This little girl was now deprived of her daily mealtime and bedtime routines, like the bubble bath at the end of each day. The rituals and schedules of Payson 7 were dictated by the need to cleanse her wounds and prevent infection. Now her "bath" would be in the morning, not the evening, and it would take place not in a bathtub but in a stainless steel tank. Janice no longer slept under her pink teddy-bear baby blanket, but in a cocoon of protective bandages streaked with Silvadene. Her dressings were decorated with protruding wires and catheters that connected her to the computer monitors that registered her vital signs. Her external defenses against bacteria were enhanced by the Silvadene, her internal metabolic supplies were supplemented by nutrition, and her mother was allowed to hold her for only a few minutes each day.

5:30 A.M. During morning rounds the staff surrounded Janice's crib. We listened to her heart and lungs with our stethoscopes, reviewed her flowcharts and laboratory results, and discussed the day's treatment plan. The burn unit doctors were surgeons, or resident surgeons-in-training—medical school graduates receiving specialty training in intensive care and trauma care under the direction of surgery professors and "attending surgeons." I was the second-year resident on Janice's team, which also comprised an intern, one year junior to me in the training program; a senior resident, two years ahead of me; and a fellow, also two years my senior. The attending surgeons, doctors whose training was completed, were responsible for supervising the entire team, and for all medical decisions on the burn unit. But the real work of hands-on patient care was done by the nurses and the residents.

The residents worked in 36-hour shifts, followed by 12 hours off; shifts began at 5:30 a.m. Every other weekend they were "on call," meaning that they reported to the burn unit Friday morning at 5:30 and worked until Monday evening at 5:30, or until all the day's work was done. Weekends off began after work on Friday. Resident rotations through the burn unit lasted for one month, long enough for the fatigue to permeate your bones. The on-call resident worked, ate, and slept (if sleep was possible) in the burn unit. A small room adjacent to the nursing station was furnished with a desk, cluttered with medical records awaiting dictation, a table usually strewn with boxes of Chinese food in varying states of preservation, a pink plastic-covered couch, and a cot. It smelled like a stale locker room. Sleep was interrupted frequently, whenever a patient took a turn for the worse, or a new admission, still smelling of smoke, arrived on the unit.

The work plan generated on morning rounds was dutifully transcribed as the "scut list," recorded by the intern, the most junior doctor on the team, who was responsible for seeing that every item on the list was completed by afternoon rounds. "Bed 16: Change IV. Bed 6: Burn wound biopsy, left thigh. Bed 2: Check blood culture and sensitivity; change antibiotics. Bed 32: Request nutritional consult." The scut list essentially outlined what everyone would do for the next 12 hours—whose turn it was to go to the operating room, and who would stay behind in the burn unit performing the patient care tasks that filled the days, most nights, and sometimes the full 36-hour shift.

10 A.M. Janice took her first trip to the "tank," a stainless steel table with walls, like an old-fashioned tub on legs, complete with drainage holes and a built-in handheld shower fixture. Under a steady stream of water from the sprayer, like the one you find on a kitchen sink, the nurses and nurse's aides gently peeled away the bandages and irrigated the burned, damaged tissue. This washed away the dead, bacteria-filled tissues and promoted healing of the deeper tissues underneath. Recalling the day my 18-month-old daughter cried in the bathtub after I gently and carefully removed a small Band-Aid from her knee, I cannot comprehend what the tank must have meant to Janice. Each time she went to the tank, the nurses pulled off 25 feet of gauze dressings from her burned arms and legs as she lay there under a steady stream of warm water. To blunt her pain and prevent her from remembering the horror of the event, we gave her ketamine, a rapid-acting anesthetic that produces a dreamlike trance. The drug's effect was to dissociate the patient from reality, creating an alternate universe in the mind, one that mercifully blocked any memory of the tank. These trips would occur every Monday, Wednesday, and Friday for the duration of her stay in the burn unit. As the bandages were removed one by one, the eschar and coagulated tissue adhering to them would be peeled off and washed away. This debridement, or removal of dead tissue, limited the available sites for bacterial growth and stimulated the growth of new tissue. Each trip to the tank required up to two hours to remove the dressings, wash the burn wounds, and reapply the Silvadene and clean sterile dressings.

A sedated Janice returned to her room from the tank. Awakening, she looked at the staff with her inquisitive eyes, as if to ask "Where am I and where are my parents?" Her family was always close by, either at her bedside when they could be, or standing down the hall between visiting hours. When it was time to go, they would lean close to her face, whisper in her ear, and hold back their tears. Outside her room, while tearing off their paper clothes, the tears came more freely, and they wondered if they would see her alive again, whether she would survive another night, whether she could feel how much they loved her, and if their presence had helped to ease her pain. Shock mingled with disbelief. The next hurdle would be an operation to remove as much of her burned eschar as possible and replace it with skin grafts. Monday, in the morning, there would be surgery.

three

The OR

Surgery to the surgeon is like a drug to an addict: under the influence, the outside world ceases to exist. The din of reality is annihilated by the smell of the mask, the warmth of the light blue sterile gown, and the pinching snap of the thin brown latex gloves. You operate automatically in a cocoon, completely engrossed and consumed by the silent checklist running in your mind's teleprompter. This trance is essential. The motions of your hands are merely the neural projections of your working brain, the result of countless rehearsals in medical school and surgery residency. Time and all bodily functions are suspended; there is no hunger, no thirst, no fullness of the bladder. All is provided for here—you desire nothing, feel nothing, and succumb to the euphoric buzz of solitude. When it is through, the skin "closed" and the bandage applied, reality returns like a slap on the face. It is painful, like being rudely awakened from a lazy Sunday afternoon snooze by the squeal of a neighbor's leaf blower.

The pager blares with a sound that hurts your ears; your head pounds migrainously as you call the answering service for your messages; nausea rises as you write the lengthening list of callbacks. Surgery is addictive, and very soon you are craving another fix. "When is my next case?" you blurt out to the scheduling manager at the OR nursing station. "Is the room clean yet? Have they sent for the patient? What is it anyway—a gall bladder, a brain tumor, or a burn?" Your insides writhe as the time passes, and you crave chocolate and caffeine to fend off the symptoms of withdrawal. Some of the more industrious surgeons run off to their offices or go to the ward, performing useful work. But many choose to wait it out in the lounge. The mood there is boisterous and upbeat, as you and your fellow addicts in the holding pen buck each other up with forced joviality during the seemingly interminable wait between cases.

The inmates in the lounge nibble on their snacks and sip their steaming cups, trying to stave off the desolate, empty feeling that comes after the intraoperative high has crashed. This stifles the painful urges but fails to produce the intense high. The discussion here is always banal and comedic; no other decorum shows proper respect to the internal longings of the participants or to the goings-on in the ORs just through the wall. Finally, they call you; the OR is clean, the patient is asleep, and you are needed.

MONDAY, MAY 6, 1985, 7:30 A.M. Janice's OR was hot—the thermostat was set to 84 degrees Fahrenheit—a necessity when the patient is a burned child. Skin is your body's insulation; it retains heat and maintains body temperature within the narrow range compatible with life. As you sit reading this book your brain is constantly sending signals to your blood vessels, adjusting the amount of blood flowing to your skin. On hot days, there is more blood flow to the face, scalp, hands, and feet, which dissipates some of the core body heat. On cold days, blood is diverted away from the skin and dermal fat layers, an efficient way to retain body heat in the deeper tissues and maintain core body temperature. Severe burn injury disrupts all that, because the fat layer in the skin, the nerves to the skin, and the associated blood vessels have all been destroyed. The burned tissue fails to retain body heat, and hypothermia quickly sets in. General anesthesia makes matters even worse, because it impairs the body's ability to regulate heat loss. Body temperatures routinely fall under anesthesia, even in patients with normal skin and an intact layer of fatty insulation. Heating blankets are used to keep anesthetized patients warm. But in burned children, like Janice, the heating blanket is not enough to keep them warm, so the entire room is warmed like an incubator.

By the time Janice was wheeled into the room at 7:45, everyone was perspiring profusely. The scrub nurse, attired in a green surgical scrub top and matching green scrub pants, had already wrapped herself in a sterile outfit of light blue paper—a gown, cap, and mask—and brown latex gloves. She extracted the surgical instruments from a stainless steel tray and arranged them neatly on a stainless steel table. The instrument table, draped in a light blue paper tablecloth, stood about four feet high and would soon be rolled into place beside the operating table. The instruments had been baked in an autoclave, a refrigerator-size pressure cooker that uses superheated steam to burn off microbes. For the remainder of the surgery, only the scrub nurse or surgeons in operating costumes would touch these instruments.

Janice had received a mild sedative for her transport to the OR, and she was dozing lightly as we lifted her from the stretcher onto the operating table. The anesthesiologist applied the "sticky pads" to her forehead and shoulder blades, connected these to colored wires with alligator clips, and turned on the cardiovascular monitor. It came to life beeping and blinking a display of her electrocardiogram. To us, Janice's heartbeat was like an announcement: "The proceedings have officially begun." The anesthesiologist then connected her arterial catheter to a pressure transducer that continuously projected her blood pressure on a small monitoring screen, and attached an oxygen sensor to a fingertip with clear plastic tape.

Normally, Janice's awake brain would silently receive and monitor all this physiological information: blood pressure; heart rate; respiratory rate; levels of oxygen, carbon dioxide, glucose, and water; and countless other vital data. These essential life data are processed from minute to minute. If something is amiss among the incoming data, your brain coordinates the physiological responses necessary to resolve a deficiency, suppress an excess, or make whatever adjustment is required to maintain health and sustain life. This vast body of incoming information is carried along from nerve to nerve, as if by a busy telephone network. Data are integrated continuously in the subconscious domains of the brain, processed, and referred to outgoing centers that communicate with the body organs and set in motion the signals necessary to maintain a balanced internal milieu.

Like any patient under deep anesthesia, Janice had ceded these regulatory jobs to the anesthesiologist. Because the drugs he would use to anesthetize her would also suppress the ability of Janice's brain to perform its regulatory role, he had to assume responsibility for her internal functions. The probe on Janice's fingertip would measure her blood oxygen level— called the oxygen saturation—by detecting the redness of the blood in her capillaries. It was critical that the anesthesiologist maintain her oxygen saturation at 95 to 99 percent at all times, because decreased oxygen levels cause brain damage. Normally of course, a probe was unnecessary, because Janice's brain constantly monitored her oxygen saturation and adjusted her heart rate, respiratory function, and even her behavior to maintain the delivery of oxygen to her tissues.

As I write these words on a yellow legal pad, I am sitting on the porch of a beachfront house on the Connecticut shoreline, gazing at three fishing boats anchored about a mile offshore adjacent to a reef formed by a sunken freighter. Schools of fish swarm the reef, their nervous systems attracted by the smaller, edible life-forms teeming around the shipwreck. Each tiny fish brain continuously reacts to the blood levels of oxygen and carbon dioxide. An unlucky fish impaled on an angler's hook is suddenly jerked shipside and onto a sunbaked hot main deck where its gills cannot extract enough oxygen from the atmosphere, or expel carbon dioxide. As the fish out of water suffocates, its brain detects the plummeting levels of oxygen and rising levels of carbon dioxide and screams emergency orders to the musculoskeletal system. The dying animal thrashes and beats with its tail, in a frantic and massive effort to leap back into the sea and swim away from the asphyxiation. Its eyes bulge; the tail and fin muscles tire; it slides deeper into oxygen debt; and then the fish brain itself fails, and the creature is dead.

It seems such a simple thing, really—you are almost never aware of it—but every second of every minute, your brain is monitoring your blood oxygen levels and responding accordingly. While the results almost never make it into your consciousness, if you were to become trapped underwater or develop a serious pulmonary illness such as asthma, you would be aware that the need for air is all-consuming, overpowering, and fundamental. Bringing a fresh gulp of air into your lungs usually passes unnoticed because your subconscious brain is in charge, quietly running the show without your conscious input, or care.

Once anesthetized, Janice's brain would be longer respond to either internal or external stimuli. She was not and would not be aware of any sudden need for oxygen; from now on, during the surgery, this was the anesthesiologist's job. He had to maintain Janice's blood oxygen levels in a safe range. General anesthesia had numbed her brain, and she would be unable to respond if her oxygen saturation fell or carbon dioxide rose to dangerous levels. If oxygen saturation were to fall during surgery—perhaps from a mechanical problem with the respirator, or because of an internal problem with the heart or lungs—there would be no brain-directed response, no leaping or flapping to alert everyone to an impending disaster, no way for Janice to climb off the table, run into the hallway, and grab a quick breath of cool air.

8:30 A.M. The anesthesiologist injected a syringe full of anesthetic into the intravenous line, and within 30 seconds Janice was deeply unconscious. Drug-induced general anesthesia is deeper than any normal sleep because the anesthetic medications stun nervous activity in the brain. Anesthesia is very unlike sleep; though the nerves residing in the brain remain alive and well, they can no longer transmit or receive information from their surroundings. There is no dreaming, no eye movement, no pleasant rolling and shifting about. The life-preserving and coordinating functions of the brain—which are largely intact during your nightly rest—are impaired during anesthesia. Drugs disable the neural networks that are the essence of your conscious, thinking, and responding brain. Major neural pathways that connect one brain region to another, and to the organs outside the central nervous system, are shut down. Communication from the command-and-control center ceases. Janice's every breath had become uncertain: high levels of anesthesia even suppress the nerves that drive the diaphragm to inflate the lungs.

The muscles in Janice's mouth and soft palate fell limp, obstructing airflow through her now collapsed airway. The anesthesiologist inserted a plastic endotracheal tube the width of

Janice's thumb down her throat and skillfully guided it between her vocal cords in order to keep her airway unobstructed. He connected the tube to a black "Ambu bag," a balloonlike device, and squeezed a few puffs of oxygen into her lungs, listening with a stethoscope for the breath sounds on each side of her chest. Then he attached the endotracheal tube to the respirator and switched on a mixture of the anesthetic gas (halothane) and oxygen. The respirator settings were adjusted—pressure, volume, and respiratory rate—based on Janice's age and size. Now, even as her deepest brain centers lay stunned and paralyzed, the anesthesiologist's respirator would provide air to her lungs.

General anesthesia has become commonplace in the modern medical system, even for children, but it is certainly not without risks. In the mind's eye of each person in Janice's operating room was a very private collection of surgical misadventures. Mistakes are integral to this process, part and parcel of the career choice. Together, this group had been exposed to or experienced dozens of "human errors" in surgery. They had heard and talked about thousands more, often in the relative safety of a "morbidity and mortality" conference, a weekly educational meeting held to review surgical complications. These conferences were integral to the education of the surgeon and the anesthesiologist.

Accidents and mistakes mold and shape medical practice intimately; practitioners at all levels of training gain experience and learn by observing the results of their own actions, and inactions, and those of their colleagues, in and around the operating room. Sometimes the deviations are minor and quickly forgotten. Others can never be forgotten—deviations so blatant that lives, of both patients and surgeons, are changed forever. Though it may seem like a basic, simple, and obvious point, Janice, like all surgery patients, had to be kept deeply asleep during the surgery, but even this seemingly simple task can go wrong.

Mikey, for example, awoke during surgery. He was 6 years old when he was accidentally shot in the abdomen at point-blank range by his older brother while they were playing with their father's loaded 12-gauge shotgun. Over a span of four years Mikey had survived 15 operations to repair the buckshot damage that punctured and shredded his bowels. The sixteenth surgery was a marathon, lasting 12 hours. At about 11 a.m., three and a half hours into the operation, the surgeon noticed that Mikey's blood had begun to ooze more freely than before, and that the bowel tissues had suddenly become pale. At the same time, the anesthesiologist noted a rise in blood pressure and increasing blood acidity. This went on for about 90 minutes, until another anesthesiologist arrived to give the first one a lunch break. On surveying the scene, he immediately noticed that the anesthesia gas had been turned off at the source. Mikey was under the knife, completely awake.

He had been unable to move because he had received high doses of paralytic drugs to keep him still during the surgery. I was a student observer, scrubbed and gowned, and holding a retractor on his intestines. I went to visit him afterward and stood at his bedside with my mouth gaping as Mikey recounted for me the specific content of conversations that had occurred during his surgery. He repeated the technical jargon word for word and vividly described the nursing change of shift that had occurred midway through his surgery. I knew he was correct, because I had been there, heard the conversations, and seen the nursing shift change. He even wondered whether one of the scrub nurses had made it through the rush-hour traffic in time to meet her fiancé at a local restaurant that evening. He accurately reported not only the discussion topics but the individual speakers. He told me that the surgeon's two hands manipulating his intestines inside his open abdomen felt both painful and nauseating. I uneasily recalled holding the retractor that tugged on his intestines. I told him that the stress he had experienced had caused temporary abnormalities in his blood clotting and acidity and blood pressure. All these changes had normalized when the replacement anesthesiologist discovered the problem and switched the anesthesia on again.

Janice did not awaken during her surgery; she remained asleep throughout her operation—safely, deeply asleep. Her anesthesiologist provided for her every breath, and gave enough sedation to prevent her from forming any memories of the surgery. Lying asleep now on the operating table, with the endotracheal tube protruding from her mouth, Janice looked like a small, doll-size mummy that had been desecrated by vandals. Her wrappings were white, but dirty and splotched with black streaks in places where the Silvadene had oozed through the gauze. In the hot room, musty, pungent odors of burn wounds and Silvadene planted themselves at the back of our noses and throats—a combined stench not unlike a sticky, sultry, festering swamp. At least the smell was not as bad as flame-injured skin, which combines the stink of sulfur and singed hair. The respirator cycled rhythmically, moving air in and out of Janice's lungs and causing the dressings over her chest to rise and fall once every five seconds, as if the dressings themselves were breathing for her. Perspiring, we unwrapped Janice's bandages to reveal the ugliness beneath: injured tissue that was dry and white in some areas but weeping, red, and wet in others.

The nurses and doctors working in those unpleasant surroundings had made a series of fundamental choices placing them squarely on a path to that place and time. Only one person in the room had not in one way or another chosen to be there—Janice. It is always that way, I suppose. No one volunteers to be burned, or decides during a morning shower that today is a good day to feel a cancerous breast lump. But accidents and diseases happen, and sometimes, as in Janice's case, the victim is powerless to stop them. Accidents can seal the fate of guilty and innocent alike. Janice's innocence and youth tugged at the hearts of the surgeons and nurses; it was not her fault that she had to suffer through all this. We discussed the plans for the surgery.

The plan for this operation was to remove eschar to uncover the healthier tissue beneath. The healthy tissue would be covered with skin grafts obtained from Janice's unburned regions. Her family, wanting to do anything they could, had offered to donate their own skin, but this was not necessary. When Janice's own donor skin ran out, we would use cadaver skin from the skin bank. Removing eschar with a knife is admittedly a crude and macroscopic substitute for the normal daily turnover of dead skin that occurs during bathing, but washing is insufficient to remove eschar. It must be cut off. Replacement skin would be shaved from Janice's unburned buttocks, which had been largely protected from the boiling water by her diaper. It was a dismal discussion, because we would be forced to cover more than half her wounds with cadaver skin, which would not heal permanently like her own donor skin. Cadaver skin is a temporary fix, a biological dressing that covers the excision and facilitates blood vessel growth in the deeper tissues. Later, however, after her own donor sites healed well enough to be harvested again, the cadaver skin would be removed and the regions covered with her own skin.

8:40 A.M. The attending surgeon and I surveyed Janice's position on the operating table, glanced over the instruments displayed on the table, and walked outside to the scrub sink in the hallway. It is always the same: We scrub by lathering up to the elbows, never above, on both arms, then using a stiff brush to scour off the detritus, with 40 brush strokes on each finger (10 each on four sides). Then wash the palms and arms. Rinse and repeat. Rinse and repeat. Watch the detritus, germs, and soap bubbles swirl down the drain. The sound of running water and the crisp, painfully abrasive brush slows your breathing and heartbeat and soothes your brain. Upon reentering the room, I was greeted by the scrub nurse, already safely cocooned in blue paper.

She handed me a sterile towel to dry my hands, then she held open my own blue paper gown. I entered it by stepping forward with my arms outstretched. The blue paper felt cool and welcoming. She held open a sterile glove, and I stuffed one hand inside, then repeated the process for my other hand. The brown latex was snug on my fingers. Then I handed her the string attached to the front of my gown, and spun around in a quick circle; she handed the end of the string back to me and I tied myself into the blue paper. Right then, as always at this point, the tone in the room changed.

Trust me—the movies and TV shows have it all wrong. Real life is not like what you've seen performed by actors: the room is not tense; it is not dramatic; it is not suspenseful; but it is mysterious. The people holding the knives and drills and saws are dressed for work, but all you can see is their eyes. All innuendo and nuance of facial expression is restricted to a raccoon strip across the eyes. The rest is hidden by masks, hats, and gowns. Communication is muffled, the voices mingled with the rustling paper gowns. Participants in this surgical ritual only rarely make eye contact, because they are watching the incision, their instruments, their monitors, or the patient. Speech is used sparingly, issued with a special rhythm, a practiced cadence that, unlike in the movies, gives no hint of tension, no emotional information.

The movies did get one thing right. When it is time to

start—*every* time an operation gets under way—the surgeon *always* puts out a hand and says "Knife." Do you imagine the scrub nurse could possibly not know what implement is needed at that point? Could she be thinking of anything else? I doubt it. But when the word is spoken for all to hear, it gives pause to everyone in the room. For that millisecond, if they like, the participants can pretend what it feels like to be in the movies.

9 A.M. The circulating nurse had finished painting Janice with Betadine, a dark brown iodine-like antimicrobial solution that reduced (but did not completely eliminate) the bacteria on her eschar and donor skin sites. I said "Knife," and the scrub nurse obligingly slapped the instrument into my palm. Looking nothing like a scalpel or a typical kitchen blade, the instrument used to remove eschar resembles a cross between a hacksaw and a machete. Called a Humby knife, it is 16 inches long and cuts with a back-and-forth sliding motion across the burned tissue, held taut by the surgeon's assistant. A special touch is required, and you have to be careful not to cut too thickly. Once I cut off the tip of one of my assistant's fingers with the Humby—it healed fine after about six weeks, and he lost only about a week in the OR. He had momentarily forgotten his role as an assistant during that surgery. A good assistant is like a good caddy while his golfer putts: when the surgeon is cutting, it is best to be still and silent, and motionless unless directed. Unrehearsed movements are equally disastrous for the putter, the surgeon, or the assistant who repositions his fingers as the Humby moves by.

We began to excise Janice's eschar, exposing the bleeding tissue beneath. As the burned coagulum was pulled back, the knife transected tiny capillaries, arteries, and veins that began to spout little droplets of blood. The volume of each droplet was small, but the cumulative blood loss produced by the excision of a large percentage of a small child's skin can quickly become significant. Surgeons, anesthesiologist, and nurses conspired to track the blood loss. Every blood-soaked sponge was collected and weighed, and the sum was used to calculate the amount of blood that had leaked out of Janice. The weights of the sponges were carefully recorded and monitored, because there is almost no margin for error. Blood volume depletion in small children can quickly lead to stroke, heart attack, or kidney failure.

Paradoxically, the anesthesiologist removed yet more blood, an additional tube containing a teaspoon of Janice's blood directly from her arterial line, which was sent to the central laboratory for measurement of her red blood cell count. Within one hour Janice had lost 10 percent of her circulating blood volume, so the anesthesiologist ordered replacement blood from the blood bank. He started a transfusion of fresh blood, now growing a bit concerned because children have very little physiological reserve, and if they become depleted, they may suddenly go into shock. He was quiet, but busy, calculating how best to compensate for Janice's blood depletion, watching the replacement blood flowing into her veins, checking the newest red blood cell count from the lab, recording the results, and thinking through his various other treatment options and contingency plans in case something unexpectedly went wrong. Years of handling similar situations with other patients had taught him the best way to avoid repeating past errors and complications.

Thin layers of Janice's healthy skin were excised from her buttocks using an electrical appliance called a dermatome, which shaves off a layer of skin ten thousandths of an inch thin. It buzzes like a barber's haircutter, producing donor skin that is rolled out in three-inch-wide strips. These were fed into another machine, operated by turning a hand crank on the side, that converted her thin, healthy skin into a mesh that looked like chicken wire. This thin mesh could now be stretched to cover a significantly larger area than would be possible with the intact donor skin. This new skin graft would be full of small holes, but if all were to go well in the next few days, each small perforation would become the home for new capillaries and skin tufts that would grow and expand, filling the voids and covering the defects.

In removing the donor skin, the surgeon is careful to cut only partially through the thickness of the skin, preserving the deeper layers necessary to regenerate the donor site with new skin. We placed the grafts carefully onto the excision sites where eschar had been removed and a stippled pattern of tiny blood droplets decorated the surface, awaiting the new skin. The coagulating blood helped glue the graft in place, but staples were needed to secure the edges and prevent them from curling up. Then we applied a pressure dressing to stop the bleeding under the grafts: too much hemorrhage will elevate the graft from the tissue beneath, causing it to slough off, rendering all the work for naught.

We cut and pasted again and again for nearly three hours until the eschar was excised. When Janice's own supply of donor skin had been exhausted, we switched to cadaveric human skin. It was hard to touch this skin without thinking about the donor who had given this gift to Janice. Who died? How? And how old were they? I have known intimately only one medical cadaver: Mrs. G, as she was known, had donated her entire body to my medical school, and it was she who guided me through gross anatomy. We opened her up and she taught us. From her we learned how each body part is connected to the brain and heart, and how the whole complex assembly is wrapped in skin.

Mrs. G rested with 29 other cadavers on a dissecting table in a large room lit by fluorescent lights and the natural light that passed through narrow windows set high up in the wall. A powerful adjustable light was hung from the ceiling over each body. We pulled back the sheet to see Mrs. G for the first time, our nervousness mingled with gratitude for her gift to us. In life she had made the choice to assist us in learning anatomy so that we could become physicians. This room was unlike Janice's OR because the anatomy dissecting suite smelled distinctly of formaldehyde, an odor that burned the nostrils and loudly announced to our brains that Mrs. G was no longer counted among the living. Her formalin-treated cadaver skin was yellowed and thickened, coarse and leathery; indeed, the preservative and embalming chemicals had tanned Mrs. G's skin. The chemicals had cross-linked the previously flexible proteins in her skin and converted them into a meshwork of strong inelastic fibers that could have become the substance of shoes, luggage, and automobile seats.

Skin prepared for the skin bank was fresh, and not exposed to embalming chemicals. Harvested within hours after the death of some nameless and considerate donor, the skin was perforated, stretched into thin layers, packed into a sterile envelope, and frozen. Handling this gift to Janice rekindled the gratitude that I felt toward Mrs. G. Now I would pass on another donor's detritus to Janice, a precious gift to a young child in need. He (or she) was gone, but the donated skin would live on for a short while longer, wrapping Janice in a biologically active dressing that we hoped would protect her from the elements better than any manufactured dressing. A stranger's kindness provided Janice not with a new baby blanket to keep her warm and cozy but with another kind of cover, far more precious: new skin.

If Janice's surgery was successful, the perforations in the

new grafts would soon become occupied by a framework of new capillaries growing up from below. Ultimately, larger blood vessels would sprout and perfuse the injured region with a new blood supply. Incoming blood would deliver not only oxygen, glucose, and other nutrients needed to regenerate skin but also new cells that could move into the area and replicate. Stem cells might arrive via these new arteries and climb onto the tissue scaffolding, where they could take root, replicate, multiply, and grow. In the ensuing weeks the new cells would produce collagen and other proteins to replace the original scaffold that the burn had destroyed. A scar would form. Although this scar tissue would never look the same as her original skin, it would provide a biological barrier against bacterial invasion, and it would reduce heat and fluid loss. Macrophages and other cells could resume their positions on the front lines, establishing a new barrier to germs. Janice's defenses against infection would begin to be refortified.

In the next two or three weeks, most of the skin grafts from the skin bank would slough off like apricot jelly during dressing changes in the tank, where they would slip and slide down the drain. But until then they would serve a useful purpose by protecting Janice from dehydration and stimulating the growth of new blood vessels, necessary for the formation of a scar. We planned to bring Janice back to the OR as needed, repeating this process until all of her wounds were covered with her own skin, or healed.

2 P.M. The eschar had been excised, the defects covered with skin grafts, and everything swathed in Silvadene and clean white gauze dressings. The anesthesiologist switched off the halothane and stood by as Janice slowly began to awaken. The monitors indicated that her heart rate and blood pressure were on the rise. Then her arms and legs began to move, and her head started to turn slowly from side to side. The anesthesiologist decided that it was time to hand the physiological reins back to Janice's still sleepy but now functional brain. Before he removed her endotracheal tube, he made sure that Janice was alert enough to maintain her own airway, because if she was not, it would collapse, her tongue and soft palate would block her trachea, and she could suffocate. When it was time, he removed the endotracheal tube. At first she breathed comfortably into a face mask that he held over her mouth and nose. But then she began the soft whimpering cry of an 11-month-old afraid of waking up in a strange room full of unknown masked adults all dressed in blue paper uniforms.

Surgeons and nurses began tearing off their blue paper gowns, tossing them onto a growing mountain of paper clothing in the corner of the room. The green scrub shirts were wet with sweat in bands across the back and under the arms. Voices were muted and parched. The intraoperative banter and synchronized movements were already a distant memory.

It had been an exhausting, hot, and dehydrating day of surgery; our defenses were down, and we were not prepared for what happened next. Janice, coming around, was afraid, crying harder now with a sob that originated deep in her abdomen, then squeaked out softly between each breath, followed by a short rush of air inhaled through her sniffling nostrils. This painful cycle repeated over and over. We were all caught off guard by this intrusion of sincere emotional content into the previously sterile room. A nurse thoughtfully lowered her mask and began to whisper in Janice's ear, talking in those quiet, kind tones that distressed parents use in their effort to comfort an injured child.

Surprised, we hurt for Janice. Our collective immunity to her pain, though fully intact a few minutes earlier, had suddenly vaporized. Our own eyes began to fill with tears, and heads shook slightly from side to side as some of us thought that our own children could be lying in this awful place, scared and in pain. Pity, not unwelcome but not invited either, had broken the surgical spell.

Empathy changed the OR, and now everything was suddenly too real: a child burned by accident, and an anguished, worried family out there waiting to hear what had happened to their only child today. The heat; the need for a cold drink. And the brutal reality that we did not know for certain whether our efforts had successfully added time to Janice's life. Janice's reality had become ours to witness, and feel. She was no longer covered by the blue drapes, and we were no longer covered by our gowns and masks. Irrationally we think, "None of this would have been a problem if I had left my mask on." Deep denial is part of the surgical trance; it is all too easy to blame the pain on the missing disguise. Denial is a consensus mandated by the conspiring participants: pretend that nothing happened.

The surgery was completely over. With faces and eyes now fully visible, the closeness and precision of the operation were shattered. Everyone looked and sounded different. It made no sense, of course, because we all knew each other well, but conversations in the cafeteria and other "public" places were always distinctly professional, clipped, reserved, and guarded—so unlike the "private" operating room mode of communicating, veiled behind masks. Unmasked, your motions feel clumsy and awkward, a harsh contrast to the graceful activity of the surgery. Voices are strained, not smooth, as if bemoaning the absence of the security provided by the costumes. None would say it, but the participants had left their intraoperative fugue state. But before Janice was even out of the room, the nurses and surgeons were already longing for the start of the next case, for the next chance to retreat into that comfortable place in which the private conversational mode would return, picked up seamlessly and effortlessly right where it had been left off.

The masks prevent surgical infections, but they also create a safe place to hide from the patient's pain. The costumes and ritual help guide the participants into their detached state. I believe that this is a vital mechanism, honed by thousands of hours spent behind masks and paper gowns while cutting into sleeping humans, that optimizes performance and improves the odds for a patient's good surgical outcome. The disguised team works as one, communicating with verbal and nonverbal signs that focus every action sharply on the needs of the sleeping patient. The atmosphere creates a powerful sensation of belonging to something larger than yourself. On long cases you derive energy from the whole team, feeling as if they empower you to function and operate for hours without fatigue. You feel that they sustain you through the toughest challenges and misadventures: you are not alone, but working beside colleagues with whom you communicate almost subconsciously. Thus fully engaged, you also enjoy a state that removes you far from any emotional response to the patient's suffering.

Janice was calmed by the nurse's soothing, something the nurse would later say was all part of her job. Of course it was not; it was heartfelt and personal. Soothed, Janice drifted back into a light sleep. She was calm, but everyone else in the room was intensely aware of the real world, the one that had ceased to exist behind the surgical masks and gowns. There were tasks to be completed, orders for Janice's postoperative care to be written, and other patients waiting in the burn unit for us to examine, laboratory test results to check, medication orders to be written, and catheters to be changed. It all flooded into our collective consciousness as if a dam had burst. Turning toward the door, we pushed Janice back to the burn unit, to the room where her steel crib lay under the pictures of an unburned Janice, lovingly taped there by her family, from the time when she had been safe from the burn unit and the operating room. Then I went to find the family and have the talk.

They were waiting in the foyer near the elevator bank just outside the burn unit. Even years later—after thousands of such one-sided "chats"—I have never become completely inured to this process. These meetings were always difficult, even when the surgery went perfectly. Janice's mother, father, and grandmother were all there. The talk was not scripted, but it could have been. I began by explaining that the surgery was over and that Janice was awake and safe back in her room. At this point most patients would be recovering in the post-anesthesia care unit or recovery room, but since Janice was in an intensive care unit on Payson 7, equipped similarly to a recovery room, she could recover in her own room instead. I said that we had accomplished everything we had set out to do; there had been no complications. This part of the dialogue was always relatively easy and straightforward; what followed was the hard part. In cases like Janice's, the chat would inevitably culminate in the realization that, after all the stress and worry and concern, things were now largely unchanged. The same worries, fears, and uncertainties returned.

In the days before surgery, the family had imagined the worst possibilities about the surgery itself. They had been tense with worry, fearful of all the things that could go wrong, consumed with a dread that was entirely focused on the surgery and the possibility that Janice would not make it out of the OR alive. Now I was standing there telling them that the major target of their worry was over and no catastrophe had occurred: Janice was fine. But she was still the victim of a life-threatening burn, and just because she had made it this far did not mean she was ready to go home, or would ever make it home. No one knew what was going to happen next.

Then came the specific questions, the ones that lay the foundation for all the new worry that was already under construction in their minds. Could she develop new complications tonight or tomorrow? Maybe, I said; she could bleed through her grafts and need either blood transfusions or a return trip to the operating room. She could develop an infection, I said, because the surgery could stir up the bacteria, inciting them to invade her bloodstream. I explained that infection in the bloodstream could lead to shock, so we would be keeping a very close watch on her heart, kidneys, and lungs. We also had to be careful that these organs properly handled all the fluid and blood that she received during her surgery.

It went on: Do you think she will have to go through this again? When will she be able to go home? As gently as possible, I told them that she would probably have to return to the operating room for another surgery in a week or ten days, and that no one knew when she would be able to go home. Some of her skin grafts would probably have to be replaced, and some of the burn wounds that we had not excised might have to be excised and grafted later. It was impossible for me to predict when she would be discharged, because there was too much that could happen. She was still at an extremely high risk for developing a severe infection. They were crestfallen and did not want to chat anymore.

By now they had nearly forgotten their dread of the surgery—and the stress of waiting to see if Janice would make it through. It was a faded memory, blocked from their minds. The surgery had ended less than an hour ago, and I was still wearing my sweaty scrubs, but to the family it may as well have been last year. Their worry and uncertainty was back, displacing their fear of the operating room. Until now they had imagined that if Janice just made it through, they would feel so much better. I do not doubt that they experienced some minor sense of relief that the surgery had not made her worse, but it was a joyless, emotionally empty time. So, after putting on their bravest faces, they thanked me for "everything you have done for Janice," and I turned to walk back toward the locker room to change out of my scrubs. I glanced back to see them staring forlornly through the windowed door into the burn unit, catching glimpses of the various nurses, technicians, and doctors entering and leaving Janice's room. They gauged her progress by studying this activity, watching the people caring for their child outside their reach; it made them feel closer to Janice.

Walking alone down the long empty hallway, I felt tired and unsure of everything. Tomorrow would not be a better day; Janice would have to struggle to survive her first major setback.

four

Shock

Messina, Sicily, October 1347. Early in the month a tattered and diseased fleet of 12 merchant ships limped into port after a difficult trading voyage to the Black Sea. Its cargo of trading goods included the mysterious and untreatable disease that had infected the crews, carried in the fleas living on the furry black rats crowding the ships' holds. The infected *Rattus rattus* leaped from the ship and ran down the docking ropes into town, eventually transmitting to the unsuspecting townspeople an infectious disease that changed history. This was the beginning of the European epidemic known at the time simply as the pestilence, a terrifying illness that spread rapidly. From Sicily it swept into Italy, then marched northward through the Western European continent, indiscriminately killing young and old. By the time it had spread into northern Sweden in 1350, it had killed between 25 and 50 percent of the population of Western Europe—20 million people.

Some cities were harder hit than others. The city of Florence lost between 50 and 75 percent of its population in one year; Venice lost 60 percent over 18 months. At one point the death rate in the fabled city of canals reached

600 people a day. There was little the physicians of the time could do, other than console the sick and dying. Today we understand that the disease was plague, perhaps the most virulent of bacterial infectious diseases, but this knowledge did not come until 500 years after the horror of the fourteenth-century pestilence.

The fourteenth-century physicians believed Galen's theories that diseases were caused by an imbalance in bodily "humors" that traveled in the bloodstream. The major therapies of the day were efforts to restore balance by blood-letting or purging with enemas. It is likely that these treatments in many cases caused severe dehydration that probably hastened or nearly assured death. Despite their inability to cure plague victims, the physicians became quite diagnostically skilled, recognizing that the disease caused distinctly different clinical symptoms and signs in different patients.

They knew that some patients developed a slowly progressing disease that evolved over one or two weeks. This form of the disease appeared as fever, flulike symptoms, a rose-colored rash, and swollen, painful lymph nodes in the axillary regions and groin, termed buboes, which gave the name "bubonic" to this form. Painful bleeding under the skin caused the appearance of purplish lesions. Diarrhea, painful abdominal crises, and vomiting came next. Mortality rates from the bubonic syndrome were between 35 and 60 percent, with death usually following an illness lasting one or two weeks. When the disease spread to the lungs, it caused a "pneumonic" syndrome, resulting in paroxysms of cough, bloody sputum, and signs of asphyxiation, including confusion, coma, and death.

The physicians recognized another, very different form of the disease, with more acute and rapidly progressive signs and symptoms. Those stricken with this form died suddenly, sometimes within hours of the appearance of a single, tender, reddish purple pustule on the skin. This acute, "septicemic" form of the disease lasted 24 hours or less, with the sudden onset of high fever followed within hours by prostration from shock, along with discoloration of the fingers and toes, which turned gray, then deep purple black. Centuries later the term black death was coined to commemorate the necrotic blackened hands and feet that typified this form of the pestilence.

Throughout history, whenever physicians recognize that a new disease has emerged, from smallpox to AIDS, they begin by looking for common signs and symptoms of the disease. This information is cataloged as a means of placing patients into distinct clinical groups characterized by similar patterns of suffering and damage. Specific common traits are described in startling detail, guided by clinical experience and careful observation of the relevant signs and symptoms. At the heart of clinical discovery is a vivid, often lurid, description of a diseased patient that lays bare the disease's essential features and clinical signature. For years, or even centuries, subsequent clinicians compare and contrast what they observe in their own patients with the original descriptions. A "classic" first description captures the essence of a malady, as well as the key features that distinguish it from other diseases—it is timeless and accurate, from the day it is first recorded.

Consider this classic description of the plague in 1347, by Agnolo di Tura, of Siena: "The mortality in Siena began in May. It was a cruel and horrible thing . . . It seemed that almost everyone became stupefied seeing the pain. It is impossible for the human tongue to recount the awful truth. Indeed, one who did not see such horribleness can be called blessed. The victims died almost immediately. They would swell beneath the armpits and in the groin, and fall over while talking. Father abandoned child, wife husband, one brother another; for this illness seemed to strike through breath and sight. And so they died. None could be found to bury the dead for money or friendship. Members of a household brought their dead to a ditch as best they could, without priest, without divine offices. In many places in Siena great pits were dug and piled deep with the multitude of dead. And they died by the hundreds, both day and night, and all were thrown in those ditches and covered with earth. And as soon as those ditches were filled, more were dug. I, Agnolo di Tura . . . buried my five children with my own hands. . . . And so many died that all believed it was the end of the world."[3]

Another description was written in the fourteenth century by the surgeon Guy de Chauliac: "It was of two kinds: the first (outbreak) lasted two months, with continued fever and expectoration of blood. And they died of it within three days. The second was, all the rest of the time, also with continued fever and apostems and carbuncles[4] on the external parts, principally in the armpits and groin, and they died of it in five days. And it was of such great contagiousness (especially that which had expectoration of blood) that not only in visiting but also in looking at it, one person took it from another: so that the people died without servants and were interred without priests." De Chauliac then developed the disease himself, surviving to recount his own illness: "I fell into a continued fever, with an apostem on the groin, and sick nearly six weeks, & was in such great danger that all my companions believed that I would die, but the apostem becoming mature, & treated (with cupping, scarification, and cauterization), I escaped by the will of God." For centuries the cause of the plague remained a mystery, leaving the priests, philosophers, and physicians to speculate about its origin, writing with wonderment and despair. Their prosaic descriptions of corpses lining village streets, with no one left to sit by the suffering ill as they died, or bury the dead, are horrifying, even when filtered by the passage of time.

The historical record indicates that plague outbreaks recurred for centuries afterward, spreading death from populated towns to quiet villages and boroughs, killing entire families, even entire cities. These outbreaks occurred cyclically, separated by relatively disease-free intervals of 2 to 20 years, just long enough in some cases to affect each succeeding generation, a process that would be repeated until the twentieth century. During one of the seventeenth-century pandemics a Jesuit priest, Athanasius Kircher, wondering about the then mysterious cause, took up the pen in 1680 and made vague reference to a causative toxin, writing that "the pestilential poison is driven by the heart into the liver and the rest of the body to spoil such weak and ignoble members with a harmful inflammation . . . Then the poison rages within, conquers the entire body and overwhelms him and finally brings about death."[5] The priest's remarks were prescient, made without knowledge of microbiology, immunology, or cytokines. Not for 200 years would we understand that cytokines made by the immune system in response to the plague infection caused the clinical signs and symptoms of the septicemic and bubonic syndromes.

Effective treatments for plague were not possible until late in the nineteenth century, when its cause was discovered. In 1894 two investigators, working separately, Alexandre-Emile-John Yersin and Shibasaburo Kitasato, isolated and identified the Gram-negative microbe during an outbreak of plague in Canton, China. Within days of each other, they reported their discovery of the germ that caused plague. Later investigators found some of Kitasato's statements to be contradictory or erroneous, so in the 1960s the organism was named *Yersinia pestis* in Yersin's honor. Yersin realized that the human epidemics occurred after the disease first began killing rats, a fact consistent with the now-known spread of the microbes, whereby fleas transmit the disease from rodents to humans.

The discovery of the *Yersinia* bacterium finally made possible the development of a specific and effective treatment for plague, nearly 500 years after the devastating pestilence of 1347–1350. The causative microbe was grown in laboratory incubators, killed, and used to inoculate horses for the production of antibodies. The earliest effective therapies were equine antiserums that neutralized the deadly effects of *Yersinia pestis* in patients. These antiserums significantly reduced mortality decades before antibiotics were developed for clinical use in the twentieth century. "Yersin's antiserum" saved countless lives because it targeted the specific agent that caused the disease in both its bubonic and septicemic forms. I suspect that someday our successors will look back with dismay and horror at how ill-prepared we were, at the end of the twentieth century and the beginning of the twenty-first, to treat the complications of infectious diseases in intensive care units.

TUESDAY, MAY 7, 1985, 9:45 P.M. Janice's blood pressure suddenly plummeted. She had been sleeping since about 6 p.m. What we did not realize until her blood pressure fell was that she had not been enjoying a peaceful rest but had entered a state of paralyzing stupor that would last for three days. Janice had gone into shock, an often-fatal medical emergency that occurs when blood pressure falls below the critical level required to maintain blood supplies to the organs, which, deprived of oxygen and nutrients, begin to suffer from asphyxiation.

To understand shock, consider that blood pressure levels are normally maintained within a narrow range, as each heartbeat squeezes oxygen-rich red blood into the arteries. Arteries produce resistance to blood flow, creating a peak pressure (known as systolic) in adults that is typically between 110 and 130 mm of mercury (Hg). (Children have lower peak pressures, which, depending on their age, range between 40 and 80 mm

Hg.) The higher the resistance in the arteries, the higher the blood pressure (for example, pinching a straw as you exhale through it causes a higher pressure in your mouth). The arteries are also distensible, stretching a bit with each squeeze of the heart. The tautness, or "tone," of the arteries is crucial, because if they become too rigid, blood pressure can become significantly elevated, a potentially dangerous form of hypertension. But if the arteries are too elastic, or "vasodilated," and fail to produce enough resistance, blood pressure falls, and not enough blood flows to the tissues. Like the old adage "Just enough is just right," proper blood vessel tone is essential to prevent shock and maintain blood flow.

If blood pressure falls below a critical level, leaving tissues and organs starved for oxygen, glucose, and other nutrients, the result is shock. As is the case in a heart attack, when a blocked coronary artery prevents blood from perfusing a region of the heart, or a stroke, when a region of the brain does not receive enough blood flow, during shock blood flow can be decreased to all the major organs. If shock persists for a prolonged time, it causes irreversible organ damage, as vulnerable cells die from a shortage of oxygen and glucose. The brain, kidneys, and heart are exquisitely sensitive to damage from shock and can begin to fail after even relatively short periods of low blood pressure. Prolonged periods of low blood pressure, lasting more than 30 minutes, take a severe toll on other organs, including the liver and lungs, which can also fail. If shock is not reversed and damage accumulates in several organs, it becomes quite likely that the patient will die even if the blood pressure is raised back to normal levels.

We knew Janice's fallen blood pressure was an emergency. We could almost hear her clock ticking down, each minute carrying her insidiously closer to permanent organ damage and death. Her lab results indicated that the white blood cell count had increased significantly, to 21,000 cells/mm³, as compared with her previously normal levels, 7,000 to 8,000 cells/mm³. Her platelet count fell, her blood sugar increased, and her body temperature dropped to 95 degrees Fahrenheit. This meant that Janice had developed shock as a result of an infection, a condition known as septic shock.[6] During septic shock, her arteries suddenly and inappropriately dilated, causing a significant drop in their resistance to the pumping action of the heart. This lowered her blood pressure and reduced the blood flow to her major organs to a dangerously low trickle. Making matters even worse, during septic shock both the blood and the blood vessels become sticky and prone to clotting. Janice's small blood vessels in her organs became clogged with clots, further restricting their ability to deliver life-sustaining blood. The mortality of septic shock can be as high as 40 to 90 percent, depending on the age of the patient, the severity and duration of shock, and the extent of organ damage.

Acute septic shock is a dramatic and frightening affair to witness—physicians inevitably remember with striking clarity their first case. Dr. Mitchell Fink, professor and chairman of the Department of Critical Care Medicine at the University of Pittsburgh and one of the world's experts in this syndrome, recalls: "During my first year as a surgery resident I wheeled a 77-year-old man down to the ICU. He had undergone a colectomy[7] for cancer, and was actually doing well until he developed an infection at the site of his intravenous line. His blood pressure fell so low that we could barely measure it; he became confused and stuporous. We measured his cardiac output and found that it was 14 liters per minute, a huge amount, comparable to what the heart of a marathon runner pumps during the fifteenth mile! And here he was, 77 years old with almost no blood pressure. I remember this like it was yesterday; I remember thinking that there was very little that I could do for him, because I did not understand what was going on, or why it was happening. I wanted to understand this so that in the future I could help some other patient."

9:50 P.M. Standing at Janice's bedside, I was in many ways no better equipped to deal with her disease than the fourteenth-century physician who, when faced with a patient with septicemic plague, would have wondered about the status of the humors in her blood. I knew that Janice needed fluids to stave off dehydration, but I did not know what had caused her to develop acute septic shock. We first increased the rate of intravenous fluid infusions to expand her blood volume and increase her blood pressure despite the dilated arteries. We knew she had an infection somewhere—perhaps in one of her burns, or maybe in her lungs, urinary tract, or other internal organ— but we did not know where. We sent samples of her blood, urine, sputum, and burn wound tissue to the microbiology laboratory where they were tested for the presence of a causative microbe. It was a futile exercise: all the cultures were negative.[8] In Janice's case, as in many cases of acute septic shock, an infecting microorganism was never found. Her chest X rays were "clear," with no sign of pneumonia, and there was no evidence of bacteria or white blood cells in her urine. Janice's shock worsened, however, and her room filled with doctors, nurses, X-ray technicians, respiratory therapists, and medical students.

Acute septic shock is a true medical emergency because there is little time to prevent permanent damage and death. The stakes are perhaps highest on the pediatric ward, because organ damage in a child will be magnified for decades to come. The medical response to this emergency is one of urgent, frenzied activity that the participants do not soon forget. Dr. Brett Giroir, the former chairman of Pediatric Care at Children's Medical Center, University of Texas Southwestern Medical

School in Dallas, recalls a case of acute septic shock caused by bacterial meningitis[9] in a 13-month-old girl: "Once you've witnessed a little child rolling her eyes back and going into shock, you remember it forever; it is horrifying. Laura had meningococcemia back in 1993 or 1994; I was a new attending and it was the peak time of year for meningococcal disease. She came in with fulminant disease; she had it real bad. As soon as she arrived in our ICU, she went into profound shock and arrested. It was the typical group scene: 10 doctors, 12 nurses, and a 1-year-old in the middle of this mass. The room was so packed you couldn't believe it. The EMTs in the ambulance had put in an endotracheal tube and a couple of lines, but we needed more. We gave her 200 cc/kg[10] of intravenous fluid in the first hour! In order to pump it in fast enough to keep up her blood pressure, we had to insert large central lines, 6 French,[11] and give the fluid that way, along with 5 percent albumin, lots and lots of saline, big doses of epinephrine, and steroids. This goes on for four to six hours! You've gotten 25 pages of orders; it was one nurse's job just to write it all down. You just keep going and going, hoping that after all this the kid will come back and show you some physiological stability, any sign of normalcy, needing less fluid and drugs just to stop her blood pressure from going to zero.

"All of a sudden, her hands and feet start to turn gray—first the feet and then the hands—and we all know what is going to happen next. What else can you do? Nothing. We have given her maximum preload—her tank is full—and she is already on epinephrine.[12] We could put on nitropaste, but we all know it is like a placebo at this point, and we do it just to make ourselves feel better. Then her hands and feet turn black right before our eyes. Finally her blood pressure is stable, but even if she does live at this point they will still have to amputate her hands and feet. She never opened her eyes again. She lasted like that for about a week, but then she developed another infection, probably from the bacteria in her bowel, and died."

10:30 P.M. We continued to pump fluids into Janice as fast as the intravenous lines allowed, but still her blood pressure drifted downward. Hour after hour, we poured fluids into her veins. This was a harrowing time, because there was no way of knowing whether Janice would cross the line, past the point of no return. The massive fluid infusion was necessary to prevent permanent organ damage, and death, but this approach also carried serious risks. Septic shock can cause the kidneys to fail, making it difficult or impossible for patients to eliminate all the excess fluid. Fluid can pool in the lungs, obstructing the fine meshwork of capillaries lining the air spaces, preventing air exchange, and drowning the patient in her own bodily fluids.

Janice's small room was crowded with two nurses, three doctors, a respiratory care technician, and a phlebotomist jostling for positions around the crib. Each was focused on the finest details of his or her job, hoping to find a clue that would suddenly turn this nightmare around and make her stable again. Janice, alone on this bizarre stage, was not perspiring. Her brain had activated a fever response, causing her face to become cool and clammy.

What does it feel like to be in septic shock? Although Janice could not describe it, some insight can be gained from others who survived the ordeal. Dr. Carl Nathan, professor of microbiology and immunology at Weill-Cornell Medical College, and an international authority on the molecular biology of septic shock, developed the syndrome as a complication of pneumonia: "I had been sick for several days, with fever and general weakness, but I thought it was nothing too serious until about six o'clock one evening, when I developed a high fever, severe shaking chill, and light-headedness. I walked to the emergency room, registered at the desk, and took a seat in the waiting area. My turn came and I started to get out of the chair, but then I realized that I could barely walk. The nurse had to help me onto the exam table, and then she took my blood pressure. I remember seeing this look of panic on her face, then she raced to call the resident over. He recognized me as a professor on the staff, and he was clearly worried. The next thing I knew, everyone was running around me; I could see it all, but through a haze or cloud. Although I wanted to, I could not move or speak.

"I remember one resident rubbing my chest, saying 'Hang in there,' and 'We're not going to let you go.' I tried to say, 'Don't worry, I'm fine,' but nothing came out. Later I found out that my blood pressure was barely palpable and that I was in florid septic shock. Although I could see all the events going on around me, I could not interact with my environment. There was no way to track the time, and I could not respond or move, but I could see and watch. It was amazing, really. The next day I was significantly improved from the fluids and antibiotics; my pneumonia continued to improve, and 48 hours later I was sitting in my hospital bed, working on a manuscript describing mechanisms of septic shock for publication in *Cell*."

Other septic shock survivors provide strikingly similar descriptions of a mental disconnection from their surroundings. Even patients who by profession and training are experts in shock, and know full well its deadliness, report a sensation of being far away from the "shock" and all the clinical activity. Consider the case of Dr. Scott Somers, a program director at the National Institutes of Health who oversees funding for many large research programs that study shock. He recalled: "We had a particularly violent gastroenteritis running rampant through our household. My turn was on a Friday. I was stricken with a rapidly progressive pneumonia, and had to be taken to the ER with a 102-plus-degree fever, heart rate of 155 beats per minute, rapid, shallow breathing, and blood pressure of 100/50.[13] I was delusional. I remember thinking that I had more than a simple (yet extremely painful) stomach disease, but as I got sicker and sicker from the pneumonia, I simply didn't or couldn't care.

"At the hospital I received intravenous fluids and antibiotics. This improved me enough to be discharged. I am struck by two thoughts. First, even though I have a pretty good idea of the biology of the septic shock response, it was simply stunning how fast it progressed. Second, an interesting mental disconnect occurred. The higher thought processes still went on but were not integrated with the ongoing sensory input. It was almost as if the more basic neurological functioning ignored the extra, unnecessary thought processing. When it finally occurred to me what was happening, I had essentially no time to act on my own accord to seek help. There is probably some important mind-body biology to be studied there. I recovered rapidly, although my blood pressure remained low (lower than the normal 110/65) and heart rate elevated (about 90 at rest, rather than the usual 60–65) for almost ten days. It was strange in that I really knew what was going on but was powerless to act upon it. Perhaps the higher cognitive aspects were influenced by the immune system's production of toxic molecules."

I do not mean to imply that the detachment experienced by Nathan and Somers is unique to shock caused by infection. I rather suspect that shock caused by other conditions, such as bleeding or myocardial infarction, induces a similar state of mind. Patients with these conditions also describe feelings of carefree nonchalance, as if they are floating or drifting a safe distance away. These events are usually recalled with a certain ease, or whimsy, an undoubtedly better aftereffect than long-standing psychological scars, which would have occurred if the brain had not set the mind apart from it all. To experience all the discomfort, medical care, and interventions with real-time clarity would surely be awful. It is as if the brain is at its editing job again, modifying the perception of events as a protective mechanism.

WEDNESDAY, MAY 8, 1:15 A.M. Janice was still in shock, with a high fever. She was stuporous and unresponsive. My neurological examination now indicated that her brain was essentially switched off, and we discussed the possibility that she might not make it. Her blood pressure hovered just above measurable levels, and her hands and feet had begun to turn gray. All seemed lost. We knew that if this persisted much longer, she would at best lose her hands, feet, and some of her hearing and other brain functions; at worst she would die. I found myself thinking, but never saying out loud, that maybe death wasn't necessarily the worst thing that could happen to Janice. At least she wouldn't have to suffer anymore.

To raise her blood pressure, we started infusing epinephrine, a powerful and potentially dangerous drug that stimulated the strength of her heartbeat and constricted her arteries. It raised her blood pressure and stemmed the tide of her shock, but before we could breath a collective sigh of relief, her urinary output decreased, and her kidneys failed. By 5 a.m. her breathing had become erratic, her arterial blood gases confirmed respiratory failure, and her chest X-rays showed signs of fluid accumulation in her lungs. We called for an anesthesiologist to place an endotracheal tube into her lungs, and we connected her to a respirator. By 8 she had stopped making urine, and her chances of ever leaving the hospital alive had fallen to less than 20 percent. Within the span of hours, Janice had developed acute septic shock, gone into a coma, and sustained major damage to her lungs, kidneys, and perhaps other major organs. At the time, we attributed this entire scenario to germs unseen. Like physicians in the Middle Ages, we tabulated and charted Janice's signs and symptoms, described her disease, gave it the name acute septic shock, and tried to restore the fluid imbalances it caused, all the while clueless about what had really caused it all.

Standing in the hallway with Janice's family that Wednesday, I tried to explain what had happened. I said that to the best of our knowledge she had an infection somewhere, that it had spread into her bloodstream, and that this "blood poisoning" had caused shock. This overlooked, or actually belied, the plain and simple fact that we had never obtained any direct evidence that Janice had an infection. Father Kircher, centuries before, had alluded to toxins, but in the late twentieth century all of our knowledge of microbes and hormones had not revealed the identity of any "toxins" that caused septic shock. There were no antidotes to these unknown molecules. We treated Janice with copious quantities of state-of-the-art antibiotics as part of our expensive and exhaustive effort to kill the bacteria that we presumed were breeding inside her somewhere.

No bacteria could be detected in our tests and cultures of her blood and urine, or in the biopsies of her burn wounds. We couldn't understand what had caused the sudden systemic collapse. We did know that infusing large quantities of bacteria into animals can cause acute shock and tissue injury, but it was puzzling that Janice, if she was indeed infected at all, had developed shock from at most a very small number of bacteria that we could not find. It just did not seem possible that a few stray bacteria floating around inside this child could account for her disastrous, still potentially fatal, circulatory collapse and widespread organ damage.

While she was in shock, Janice's brain remained completely shut down. It was as if she was suspended in time, unmoving, like sleeping without dreaming. Stealing a quick glance while passing her bed, a casual visitor could scarcely have distinguished Janice's appearance from that of a peacefully sleeping child. But closer inspection would have revealed that somehow everything was wrong; the essence of the child was not there, and there was no peace in the surroundings. An army of nurses, doctors, and technicians armed with intravenous tubes, needles, and bandages ministered to her, reinforced with heavy machinery, like the respirator that bellowed 16 times a minute with a dull, eerie cadence.

Janice lay in the middle of a noisy, chaotic battle zone but made no effort to interact within her environment, no effort to touch the bandages covering her burns. By this time her burn wounds were full of histamine, a powerful stimulus to itching, and her whole body was covered with bandages. Yet she did not fidget, tug at the dressings, or attempt to scratch. She just lay there. The endotracheal tube, a hard plastic tube as wide as her thumb, filled her airway, lodged snugly against the sensitive mucosal walls of her larynx. Nerve fibers in the larynx normally trigger paroxysms of coughing if so much as a tiny speck of dust or a drop of milk is inhaled. An endotracheal tube lodged within your throat would be intolerable; a split second after it was inserted you would be thrashing, coughing, and bucking like a fish on a hook. But Janice did not cough or buck against the respirator as it sent puffs of air into the tube, moving it slightly against the lining of her airways each time. Janice's deeply stuporous brain had ceased responding to its environment. Brain incapacitation occurs in nearly all critically ill patients, but surprisingly little is known about how the dysfunctional brain can affect the patient's outcome.

9 A.M. Almost as suddenly as she went into shock, Janice turned the corner and came out of it. Her blood pressure in-

creased and stabilized, and she no longer required massive amounts of intravenous fluid. Her hands and feet turned pink again. For the first time since Tuesday night, she opened her eyes, and then began to fight against the tube in her throat, bucking her chest with every respiration as she coughed and gagged. We removed the endotracheal tube, and soon after, a respiratory therapist arrived to reclaim the respirator, rolling it back out of Janice's room and down the hallway to stow it in the bowels of the hospital. We were all pleasantly stunned by the rapidity of Janice's recovery.

FRIDAY, MAY 10, 4 P.M. Janice's grandmother Cecilia was at the burn unit visiting her only grandchild. She was always telling stories. Cecilia was born in Italy and immigrated with her parents to Brooklyn shortly after World War II. Her father supported the family—his wife, three daughters, and a son—by selling fruit and vegetables door-to-door from the back of his truck. They were a deeply religious family, strictly observant Roman Catholics whose lives revolved around Sunday morning Mass and the holy days of the church calendar. At home on the first floor of a modest two-family house, they spent a large part of their time crowded together in the kitchen. The cooking secrets of generations were passed down from Cecilia's mother, who taught Cecilia and her two sisters how to prepare the traditional pastas, meats, and fish dishes served at the family's evening meal. Preparation of Sunday dinner, served at 2 p.m. every week, began Saturday morning. Cecilia's earliest memories were of standing on a chair at the kitchen table, turning the wooden handle on the stainless steel pasta machine that pressed the dough into wide, flat sheets and cut it into long strings of spaghetti, linguine, or fettuccine. Her sisters would remove the pasta from the machine and carefully drape it over a wooden rack, where it hung to dry in the open air.

The vegetables were fresh from the farmer's market by way of Cecilia's father's truck. Broccoli rabe was steamed, then sautéed in olive oil with garlic. Eggplant was sliced paper thin, layered on a wide screen placed over the sink for four hours so that the bitter juices could drain away, and dipped in flour, beaten eggs, and bread crumbs before it was fried in olive oil. Peppers were fried with onions, garlic, and sausage sliced on the diagonal. Tomatoes were squeezed first by hand and then pressed through a mill directly into the "Sunday gravy pot," cooked over a low flame and stirred every 10 to 15 minutes for hours until the gravy was perfect. Soon after her eighteenth birthday, Cecilia married her high school sweetheart. They moved into a three-bedroom flat, ten blocks from her childhood home, where they raised two girls and two boys. It was a large family for a small home, but Cecilia was always comfortable in the kitchen. The more crowded the better. She was happiest when her kitchen was full of family, warmed by the heat from the oven and stove-top burners. She moved quietly through the commotion caused by cooking with her two sisters and their friends, brushing shoulders, trading gossip, and keeping current on the neighborhood news.

Janice was her first grandchild, born on Cecilia's birthday, a coincidence that conferred a closeness between them beyond even that which attended Janice's status as the first. Cecilia always smiled when she said that "Janice was the best birthday present I ever had." Janice's arrival could not have been better timed. Cecilia's husband had died suddenly two years earlier, and only Janice's family had stayed nearby. The rest of Cecilia's children had moved to distant cities. Cecilia had grown lonely and frustrated by the quiet life of her newly emptied nest. Janice's parents both worked full-time, and they welcomed Cecilia's offer to watch Janice on workdays until she was old enough for preschool. Janice became the centerpiece of Cecilia's life.

After the accident Cecilia waited in the hospital all day long, and late into every night, her tired eyes lined by the dark shadows of grief, guilt, and fatigue. Standing in her yellow paper gown at the foot of Janice's crib, holding black rosary beads in trembling hands, Cecilia mumbled her prayers through the blue paper mask, sometimes in English, sometimes in Italian, begging Mary for mercy on her Janice, her most precious birthday child. Now it seemed that her prayers had been answered: Janice had pulled through her shock and was smiling at Cecilia through shining, clear eyes.

SATURDAY, MAY 11, 5 P.M. Janice's parents and grandmother hovered around her bed, smiling and kissing her face and toes, ecstatic that she had pulled through. Janice's eyes were bright as she alternately snuggled in her mother's and her grandmother's arms, emitting high-pitched squeals and chirps. It was a Saturday on the burn unit, many patients had been discharged, and there had been no admissions to replace them. Janice's 9- and 12-year-old cousins were allowed in during visiting hours, and the family began planning the festivities for her first birthday party, around two weeks away. The sun was shining, spring was in full bloom, and through the windows we could clearly see the brightly colored azaleas on the Rockefeller campus. Janice's wounds were healing better than expected, and we wondered whether she might need only one more, relatively minor, trip to the operating room. There was a great deal to be thankful for. Unfortunately, everything was to change on Sunday, when Janice first developed signs of a new complication: severe sepsis.

five

Pestilence

It is not plague but severe sepsis that is serving notice as the pestilence of the twenty-first century. Severe sepsis is one of the most common causes of death worldwide, killing nearly a quarter of a million people each year in the United States alone. Deaths from severe sepsis are eclipsed only by mortality from cardiovascular disease (930,000 deaths annually from heart disease and stroke) and cancer (556,500 deaths). Unlike the plague, severe sepsis is not contagious, but more than 4 million people have died from it since Janice's hospitalization in 1985. The number of severe sepsis deaths may actually be higher: some patients with heart disease and cancer die from severe sepsis, but their deaths are attributed to the primary or underlying disease instead. In contrast with heart disease and cancer, there are no well-funded, widely known organizations or action committees that target the disease. There is no sepsis group with the visibility and fund-raising power of the American Cancer Society or the American Heart Association.

Severe sepsis has remained below the radar of public awareness, in part because it is a diagnosis often left unspoken, even by the attending physicians, to its victims and their families. Doctors may fear its pestilential qualities more than they realize. Severe sepsis is a mysterious and un-treatable, modern-day fatal illness. It causes a protracted hos-pitalization, usually spent in an intensive care unit, where the costs can be emotionally and financially devastating.

Janice developed severe sepsis after her scald injury, but na-tionwide, burn injury is a relatively uncommon cause. The vast majority of severe sepsis cases occur in patients who are afflict-ed with more "typical" and prevalent diseases, such as heart disease, cancer, pneumonia, appendicitis, pancreatitis, chron-ic liver or kidney disease, and infections of the gastrointestinal or urinary tract, or with serious trauma from a motor vehicle accident or other injury.

The word *sepsis* comes from the Greek word *sēpsis*, meaning "decay," and *sēpein*, meaning "to putrefy," or to make rotten or foul-smelling.[14] In medical terms, sepsis is defined as either "the presence of pathogenic organisms or their toxins in the blood or tissues" or "the poisoned condition resulting from the presence of pathogens or their toxins, as in septicemia."[15] Patients are given a diagnosis of sepsis when they develop clin-ical signs of infection or systemic inflammation; sepsis is not diagnosed based on the location of the infection, or by the name of the causative microbe. Physicians draw from a list of signs and symptoms in order to make a diagnosis of sepsis, in-cluding abnormalities of body temperature, heart rate, respira-tory rate, and white blood cell count. Sepsis may be diagnosed in a 72-year-old man with pneumonia, fever, and a high white count, and in a 3-month-old with appendicitis, low body tem-perature, and a low white count.

Sepsis is defined as *severe* when these findings occur in as-sociation with signs of organ dysfunction, such as hypoxemia, oliguria, lactic acidosis, elevated liver enzymes, and altered cerebral function.[16] Like Janice, nearly all victims of severe sepsis require treatment in an intensive care unit for several days or weeks. Severe sepsis is a modern "pestilence" because, like the epidemic that killed much of Europe's population in the fourteenth century, its cause is unknown. Lacking effective treatment for the current pestilence, doctors at the beginning of the twenty-first century stand stiffly at the bedside in their white coats, and in the waiting room, speaking to the family in hushed tones while maintaining a pose of thoughtfulness and woe. Except for the modern clothing, these scenes might have come straight out of the past, as if lifted from the weathered paintings depicting professionals with concerned faces gazing sorrowfully at the victim dying of plague.

Today's doctors treat specific complications from severe sepsis as they arise. Comfort is given to patients and families; hope offered at the bedside lingers quietly, as if awaiting a promised future treatment that can effectively cure the disease. The modern pestilence of sepsis does not evoke the sheer horror of the fourteenth-century pandemic, primarily because it is not spread from house to house or town to town on the backs of rodents. Perhaps it is a less dramatic killer, but it is a common cause of death that we cannot effectively treat and are just beginning to understand.

Janice had just survived her battle with acute septic shock, a fulminant and rapidly progressing syndrome that is clinically similar to the septicemic form of the ancient pestilence. Next she would have to battle severe sepsis, similar to the bubonic form of plague. It would be a struggle that could last for days or weeks before she would either recover or die.

SUNDAY, MAY 12, 1985, 9 A.M. The pestilence of severe sepsis came upon Janice gradually in the second week of her hospitalization, not with the frantic activity of septic shock but with a grinding and prolonged assault—the kind that weakens resolve and tires the soul of patients old enough to be aware of it—a slowly burning consumption of her tissues. She spiked a 104°F fever, and the microbiology laboratory report indicated that there were microbes growing in her bloodstream. Today we understand that her fever was caused by cytokines, molecules produced by her immune cells to coordinate the inflammatory response to infection. These cytokines function as "endogenous pyrogens" to turn up the temperature set point in the body's thermostat, located deep in the hypothalamus, at the base of the brain. A moderate fever from low-level cytokine release can be beneficial, aiding the immune system's ability to kill and clear the bacteria. If cytokine accumulation in the brain becomes excessive, however, then body temperature can become dangerously high, to the point that it damages organs, including the brain itself. We gave Janice intravenous antibiotics and placed her on a cooling blanket; hoping for the best but fearing the worst, we resumed watching and waiting.

She did not go into shock, but her urine output decreased steadily throughout the day on Sunday, a sign of dehydration or kidney failure. To reverse this, we once again increased her intravenous fluid intake. Janice's face became swollen and puffy—her eyelids so engorged with fluid that they closed, blocking her view of the world. She could not see out, and we could not see in. She lapsed in and out of consciousness, sleeping almost all the time. Diarrhea developed on Sunday afternoon—a sign that her gastrointestinal tract was no longer able to absorb nutrients. We discontinued the tube feedings to reduce the dehydrating effects of diarrheal losses. Monday morning she stopped producing urine completely.

Normally the kidneys maintain a proper balance of salt and water in the bloodstream, removing and excreting toxins into the urine. One of the complications of kidney failure is potassium accumulation in the blood, a life-threatening development because elevated potassium levels cause cardiac arrhythmias and sudden death. We treated this using kidney dialysis with a portable stainless steel machine that was wheeled into her room every 48 hours. Blood was diverted from her veins into the machine, a vibrant red river flowing through clear plastic tubes that, like an umbilical cord, carried her wastes away, accompanied by a whirring, pulsing sound. Instead of her kidneys, filters and purifiers of steel and plastic balanced her potassium, keeping her alive.

TUESDAY, MAY 14, 11 A.M. Janice's arterial oxygen saturation level fell, and her chest X-ray showed diffuse lung injury. Where there should have been clear black areas depicting the air spaces in her chest, the X-ray showed white. Janice's lungs had filled with frothy fluids that looked like fluffy white clouds. To us, however, they were dense storm clouds that blackened our outlook, signaling a deadly process that blocks the effective exchange of oxygen and carbon dioxide. The normally dry spaces where the air meets the bloodstream were underwater. She was drowning in her own fluids.

Her once soft and pliable lungs were now stiff with liquid that resisted the air flowing into her lungs. Every breath was now a grueling task. Janice's respiratory muscles were tiring. Like all children, she had little excess capacity, or respiratory muscle reserve, and if she worsened much more, she might reach the point of severe muscle fatigue and simply stop breathing.

We summoned the anesthesiologist, who arrived at her bedside with his laryngoscope and assorted endotracheal tubes. Choosing the correct size tube, he slipped it in between her vocal cords and connected it to the ventilator. For the third time (once in the OR, and a second time when she was in shock), Janice's every breath depended upon the rhythmic contractions of a ventilator that pumped her lungs with a mixture of air and pure oxygen under controlled conditions of volume, pressure, and respiratory rate. We adjusted the respirator's settings to optimize the levels of oxygen and carbon dioxide in her bloodstream, then resumed our wait to see if she would stabilize.

WEDNESDAY, MAY 15, 5:30 A.M. On morning rounds we discovered that the whites of Janice's eyes were yellow; jaundice had set in. Her liver was added to the growing list of failed organs. Healthy liver cells, or "hepatocytes," produce bile and pump it into the bile ducts, which carry it to the gallbladder for safe storage. During consumption of a meal the gallbladder pumps the bile into the gastrointestinal tract, where it facilitates the absorption of fatty foods. The hepatocytes, bile ducts, and gallbladder are all impervious to bile and maintain a clear separation between the bile and the bloodstream. For Janice, as with most victims of severe sepsis, this separation dissolved, giving the bile free access to her bloodstream. The bile in her blood had increased to dangerously high levels, threatening to damage her other organs.

Once again we searched for microbes that might be causing her persistent sepsis, sending samples of her blood, urine, sputum, and burn wounds to the laboratory for testing, but none of these cultures revealed germ culprits. As best we could tell, the antibiotics had done their job and eradicated the bacteria that started this process. There were no more bacteria to be found, yet her severe sepsis was nonetheless getting progressively worse before our eyes.

Life begets toxins. Regardless of the size of the organism, whether a single bacteria, a society of 200 million people, or an 11-month-old child, survival depends on successfully compartmentalizing waste, preventing it from mingling with and poisoning the organism with its own pollution. For verte-brates, health is possible only when the vital organs efficiently eliminate the toxic wastes normally produced as metabolic by-products of cellular work. Using a grading system wherein an organ receives an A for properly doing its job—handling dangerous toxins and keeping them away from the bloodstream—Janice's kidneys, lungs, bowels, and liver each received an F. Normally the lungs handle carbon dioxide; the kidneys, potassium and excess nitrogen; the intestines, bacterial debris; and the liver, bile. Now each of these organs was either obstructed or leaking, and the waste products were building up inside Janice. Unless these conditions were reversed, she would die from the combined effects of accumulated toxins and secondary infections caused by bacteria leaking through her bowel wall into her bloodstream.

Janice's bout with the modern pestilence has similarities and differences with the ancient epidemics. A jarring similarity is that in both cases the underlying cause was not known, so the modern physicians were compelled, like their fourteenth-century predecessors, to expend tremendous efforts in defining and characterizing clinical signs and symptoms. A major difference between severe sepsis and the historical plague is that severe sepsis can develop after infection with an array of bacteria, viruses, or fungi; plague is caused by infection with one bacterium, Yersinia pestis (the bacterium that caused the fourteenth-century pestilence). Yersinia infection occurs sporadically today, in the United States and elsewhere, but it is a highly unusual cause of the severe sepsis syndrome. Other microbes are a much more common cause of the severe sepsis we encounter in our modern intensive care units. It can be caused by bacteria such as Staphylococcus aureus, Streptococcus pyogenes, Escherichia coli, Pseudomonas, and Enterobacteriaceae. Importantly though, nearly half the time, a specific infecting organism is never found, even when one is sought with advanced diagnostic tests, biopsies, and cultures. Physicians in the intensive care unit know severe sepsis when they see it—they are adept at defining its severity and prognosticating outcomes—but often they can only speculate about its cause in an individual patient.

Clinicians and scientific investigators interested in severe sepsis have spent an inordinate amount of time diligently working on a broadly accepted definition of the syndrome. They placed an extremely high premium on this, spending years debating the criteria that establish the diagnosis in an individual patient. You may wonder, fairly enough, what's in a name? For one thing, there is a fundamental human need to name that which we cannot tame or control. Like a hurricane or war, a named disease becomes part of the shared experience that memorializes the immediacy, the horror, the fear. It becomes communal, one event "known" by all. For another, terminology is vitally important for advancing research, serving as a medical-scientific "Remember the Alamo!" that focuses interest on the problem and raises awareness. These are critical steps toward mobilizing the significant resources needed to solve the problem.

Another reason lethal diseases must be named is to benefit patients and their families. A named diagnosis can be rolled off the tongue, simultaneously implying knowledge and removing some of the fear inherent in dying by an unknown hand. Even if the current "knowledge" about causation proves false someday, or available treatments ineffective, or both, the name of the disease will be discussed at the bedside, in the hospital cafeteria, and relayed on the telephone to concerned distant relatives. A name can be compartmentalized in the minds of the suffering patient and family, and dutifully inscribed in the medical records. The alternative of not knowing is painful, haunting, and terrifying. The history of medicine teaches that naming and describing the disease is really the first step toward developing an effective treatment.

The naming of previously incurable diseases, such as polio, tuberculosis, and plague, occurs long before effective therapies are developed. In the early twenty-first century we have progressed through the first two steps for severe sepsis: it has been named, and its clinical signs and symptoms have been defined. Patients can be categorized into clinical groups, regardless of whether they start out with a burn injury, pneumonia, appendicitis, a motor vehicle accident, or cancer. Its victims develop similar, overlapping clinical signs and symptoms. You don't have to be medically trained to tell the difference between a patient pulled from a car wreck with broken legs, and one admitted to the emergency room with fever and cough from pneumonia, at least not for the first few days or hours after the injury or infection. But after another week or so, if both patients develop severe sepsis, then a very different picture emerges. Now it will become difficult or impossible for you to distinguish these patients by clinical signs alone. After two weeks of severe sepsis, they will look eerily similar, lying still in their ICU beds, connected to a respirator and countless other pumps, monitors, and machines. As long as the casts on the broken limbs remained covered underneath the blankets, it will be almost impossible for you to tell which patient started with broken bones and which with a fever and cough. Severe sepsis looks like severe sepsis, and now Janice had it bad.

THURSDAY, MAY 16, THROUGH FRIDAY, MAY 24. Day after day, Janice lay motionless and swollen, kept alive by machines that breathed for her, cleansed her blood, and pumped fluids and antibiotics into her veins. This was possible only because of the nurses who watched her every minute and tended to her every need. The nursing care of a patient with severe sepsis is monumental. When that same patient also has extensive burn wounds that need hours' worth of dressing changes daily, it is overwhelming. Janice's nurses were members of a tightly knit group who were passionate in their dedication to provide the best care for the critically ill patients in their charge. At shift changes the exiting staff left the unit in groups of two or three, occasionally stopping together for a coffee or drink on the way home. They helped each other decompress from the stress— a new patient with particularly horrifying wounds, or a longer-term patient who suddenly took a turn for the worse, like Janice.

The shift replacements passed through the burn unit with confidence and pride, like airline pilots striding past their passengers waiting to board the plane. These nurses were proud, dedicated to the physically and mentally difficult work they had chosen. They were empathic to the pain of patients and the anguish of families, but the cost was a very high burnout rate. The half-life of staff on the burn unit was only about two years, so every month new faces appeared, eager to learn how to change a burn dressing, work the tank to clean the burn wounds, and treat the complications of severe sepsis. The few long-term nurses had learned how to steel themselves against the pain, or accept it, in a way that did not preclude empathy and compassion. Though their little pediatric patient lay still in her crib, unresponsive to the commotion around her, the nurses talked to Janice, pattering on as if the dressing change or trip to the tank was just another diaper change or bedtime bath at home. Because of her severe sepsis, Janice was once again unresponsive to the nurses' voices and activity. It was as if she had become disconnected from the pain and suffering here in the burn unit, and floated off to a different spot.

The nurses held Janice whenever they could, careful not to dislodge the endotracheal tube, intravenous lines, arterial line, or Foley catheter. They rocked her, sang to her, and nurtured her with a kindly touch. They hurt because Janice—and all their other patients—hurt, and when the accumulated pain got to be too much, they arranged for a transfer to another floor, one where the mortality rate, nursing intensity, and stress were significantly less. That meant any other floor in the hospital.

What does it feel like to have severe sepsis? David Sheehan, a resident of Highlands Ranch, Colorado, is a former CEO of a long-term-care organization and a survivor of severe sepsis. He recalls: "I was admitted to the hospital on September 3, because of a bowel obstruction, with vomiting and abdominal pain. They tried to get me back in shape with intravenous fluids and a nasogastric tube, but I did not get better and they had to operate on me twice. The first time was September 6, but I still hadn't improved by September 18, and they took me back in. In the recovery room that day my heart was racing at 130 beats per minute, and I was in more pain than can be imagined. They would ask me to rate my pain from 1 to 10, and I said 100. They had put a spinal needle in my back, and my stomach was hurting beyond belief. I don't remember everything, but [my wife] later told me that I said I did not want to go on if it had to be with this pain.

"From recovery I went to the ICU, where I developed severe sepsis that lasted the next eight days. I was in a sort of private room in there, my own space, but it was a surreal experience. Things happened around me through a gray haze. Some nights I would ask the nurse why they had moved me to Boulder from Littleton; of course, I had not been moved at all. My friend brought in a CD of John Michael Talbot, a monk who plays beautiful guitar music, but I made them turn it off. I couldn't listen to it because it was all out of sync—it sounded like noise, not music. I guess it was emblematic of how I related, or couldn't relate, to the world. My memories from the whole time are like a series of stills—not a movie—just 30-second-interval shots. The rest of it: gone. I was not very hopeful; it felt like it would go on forever, me suspended there between life and death, floating, not getting better, not getting worse, unable to sleep, incredibly anxious. It was awful not being able to be in one of those places or the other. I had been through many other surgeries, but I had never not known where God was. Despite my deep faith, I couldn't pray. I did not seem to know how—like with the CD, it was all out of sync.

"When the severe sepsis resolved I was sent out to a bed in a regular hospital room, and I could start to remember things, and I could pray, at first with the chaplain's help. I struggled with the meaning of the entire hospitalization, finally resolving that the adhesions that triggered it were metaphors for adhesions in other aspects of life that were keeping me from being all I could be in God's kingdom here on Earth. Carrying the pain of others was a major adhesion from which I had to detach to engage in life more fully. It was there and then that the sounds from the Talbot CD were wonderful! Its first song, 'God Alone Is Enough,' touched me deeply. It still resonates today."

The essentials of your humanness dwell in your brain. With it you think, speak, write, paint, appreciate the symmetry in fine music and art, understand your fit into the world, believe in God, and pray. It is a startling fact that if, like David, you found yourself lying in an intensive care unit bed with severe sepsis, your brain dysfunctional in a major way, your confused state would not incite an army of doctors and nurses to near-riotous activity. If, however, you were to develop a comparable degree of dysfunction in your kidney or heart, then by God, watch out! Get out of the way! They would circle your kidney or heart, pouncing quickly and assuredly with their drugs, machines, needles, tubes, and other interventions all carefully designed to rehabilitate and revitalize your failing organ and all its shortcomings. But if your highest-functioning organ, the brain in your head, that ultimate pride and joy of the human species, failed, what would happen? In a word, not much.

Dysfunctional brains are as commonplace in the ICU as Foley catheters and respirators. The brain of a typical severe sepsis patient cannot appreciate music, read the *New York Times* (or any other words, for that matter), generate a prayer, or even maintain its orientation in time and space. Yet the dysfunction, in and of itself, prompts no frantic racing about, elicits no specific intervention to support the brain's failing or restore its function. That is not to say that the physicians and nurses will not make an effort to identify a potentially reversible or treatable cause of confusion, like acute hypoglycemia, or oxygen deficiency in the blood. If they fail to find such a cause, however, the default position is to watch, wait, and see whether brain function returns on its own. Put quite simply, no one understands how the brain works, so modern medicine offers precious little in the way of "fixing it" when it breaks.

One reason the brain plays a role in severe sepsis is that technological advances in the intensive care unit since Janice's hospitalization now prolong life beyond what could previously have been imagined. This development has enabled severe sepsis to be identified, defined, studied, and categorized as a distinct clinical entity. Before the modern era of large intensive care units, in which organ function is individually monitored and maintained, patients with severe sepsis simply died of dehydration, rapidly progressive secondary infection, and the accumulation of metabolic, immunological, and bacterial toxins. Now, in ways that were impossible before respirators, death is held at bay. Some large ICUs house 50 or 60 people at a time, all of whom are dependent on the mechanical cycling of air into and out of their lungs because they have ceased breathing on their own. Dangling over the precipice, they are tethered by plastic tubing that binds their lungs and kidneys to machinery, anchoring them to the hospital and preventing their plummet into the abyss.

Our early ancestors could not have survived beyond the initial phases of severe sepsis. The afflicted would lie in their cave, perhaps arranging their affairs (if they could) before lapsing into unconsciousness from dehydration and then dying. When breathing stopped, life was over. Even as recently as the early twentieth century, the most advanced medical treatments could not support organs once they failed. Only within the past 20 to 30 years has intensive care medicine advanced to the stage at which severe sepsis patients can be supported and maintained for weeks—at a staggering cost, of course—as much as $30,000 a day or more in 2004. Patients are kept alive longer, but at the heart of the matter is a big problem—we do not know the underlying cause of severe sepsis. Future historians, looking back at the mortality rates of severe sepsis today, may well conclude that our ability to treat severe sepsis has advanced but little since the fourteenth century.

Progress for Janice ceased. Every day was the same. Wretched monotony for the family, nurses, and doctors. With nothing changing, every day slowed to a crawl. Medical news was transmitted to the family, but it lacked meaning or sense to the participants in the waiting game. Time passed but provided no context. There were no reference points, because the scenery and the script were always the same. The routines were invariant, from morning rounds to the arrival of the lab results to the dressing and line changes, followed by afternoon rounds, visiting hours, and then night rounds. Despite the danger and uncertainty, it was almost boring for its lack of variety—like an ancient water torture dripping onto the foreheads of all the participants. Janice had severe sepsis, every day, day after day. The fight was now to prevent severe sepsis from breaking the collective will of the staff to carry on. At a primitive or subconscious level, the family knew this. They sensed that this was a fight to the death, and they did all they could to buck up the troops, worrying that Janice could become a casualty in the midst of all this boredom. They were frustrated and confused about the lack of progress and by the inability of this hugely expensive and complex medical process to alter Janice's clinical course as she spiraled like a vortex in a drain, on a course that seemed headed toward failure.

Nowadays hospitals have gone to extraordinary lengths to provide some comforts for the patients' families, but this was not the norm in 1985. Janice's family had no luxuries while they waited out the storm of severe sepsis. There were no carpeted, warmly lit waiting rooms graced with a coffee machine and a TV on the wall, like those you find outside today's ICUs and ORs. Janice's family stood in a dark, stagnant nook adjacent to the two elevators around the corner from the windowed door. Sometimes I found them sitting on the floor, backs to the wall, dozing fitfully. They took turns going to the cafeteria, always leaving at least one person behind near the elevator in case a doctor or nurse came out with some news. At shift changes and lunch breaks the staff would stand waiting for the elevator, chatting with the family. The conversations always ended with Cecilia expressing her profound gratitude to us, saying through her tear-filled eyes, "Thank you so much for all you are doing for my little Janice." Visiting hours lasted ten minutes every fourth hour; the rest of the time the family stood watch by the elevators.

I don't know how they, or other parents and relatives of patients like Janice, could do what they did. Janice's mother, Maria, was a secretary in the financial district. She was a diminutive woman with shoulder-length black hair that showed signs of premature graying. Dark circles under her eyes betrayed the strain of worry and sleep deprivation. Janice's father, Frankie, was a doorman at a midtown apartment building, a job well suited to his easygoing smile and quiet voice. Waiting beside the elevator, he always looked into the eyes of the nurses and doctors that happened by, searching for evidence of news about Janice, hoping to learn as much from the medical staff's expressions as from the words they used.

He did not understand most of the words, so he left the medical conversations to Maria and Cecilia. Instead, Frankie paid attention to the nonverbal forms of communication, which relayed news via a medium with which he was more familiar and practiced. He could sense when Janice was doing better by the slope of the doctor's shoulders, or the glint in the nurse's eye, but he feared seeing the involuntary tightening of muscles around the jaws and eyes, because that always meant something had gone wrong. I suppose that Maria's and Frankie's co-workers must have helped them cover their shifts at work. One of the parents was always there with Cecilia, every day, waiting for Janice. Nights and weekends they were all there together, keeping their vigil, murmuring their prayers.

A great deal has changed since then. Now, on the pediatric wards especially, a major effort has been made to provide parents as much access as possible to their sick children. Pediatric rooms have beds or reclining chairs where parents can sleep without leaving their child's side. But in 1985 the rules were different—the family could be at the bedside only during visiting hours. One can imagine how difficult the separation from their only child was for Janice's parents, but it is inconceivable to think about what it must have felt like to the scared 11-month-old. She was just a baby who wanted—needed—to be held and rocked and comforted in her mother's loving arms. Just weeks ago her parents and grandmother had luxuriated in those moments—smelling the fragrance of baby shampoo in her downy baby hair, feeling her arms and legs twitch softly as she drifted off to sleep when her bottle was empty. In the burn unit they could not pick her up on their own—the nurses had to hand their child to them. They sat waiting in a chair with open arms, under the constant gaze of medical staff worried that one of the intravenous catheters or other lines would be pulled loose during the transfer from the crib. Janice smelled different, too—no longer of baby soaps and powders but of a strange mingling of Betadine and Silvadene.

Visiting hours ended after what seemed to the family like just a few fleeting minutes. Then it was time to transfer Janice back to the nurses and her crib. During her severe sepsis Janice was extremely lethargic, seeming not to notice who was holding her or what was going on around her. I believe, but of course cannot prove, that children have benefited immeasurably by being surrounded by their loving family, and feeling their presence even when they cannot respond. I will not be surprised if we learn one day that hospital mortality rates for seriously ill children declined in proportion to greater exposure to their parents in the hospital. It may prove to be one of the great miracles of modern medicine: encouraging parents to stay close to their children.

Once a day during Janice's severe sepsis we clustered with the family at their spot outside the elevators. Wearing our paper outfits, the medical team would stand in a circle and conduct a dialogue that was frustratingly similar to discussions we had held when Janice was in shock. It went something like this: "Yes, we think that this whole mess of sepsis got started when she had those bacteria in her bloodstream awhile back, but we gave her the newest, most improved, and greatest antibiotics to ever come along the pike. They seem to have done the trick and killed all the germs. Now the good news is that we can't find any more bacteria. The bad news is that we don't understand why she should be so sick with her severe sepsis. It could be blood poisoning again. Yes, you are right, we told you the same thing about blood poisoning when she was in shock two weeks ago, and now she is not in shock . . . it must be a different kind of poison. No, we don't know where the poison is coming from this time either, we don't know what the poison is, and we don't know how to block it or turn it off. So we just have to keep watching and waiting to see if any more complications develop. We can treat complications one at a time, we know how to do that. Let's hope for the best, but we are very worried about whether she can pull through. Yes, we are doing everything that we can, but we are incredibly frustrated too. We can't imagine how hard this must be for you."

At this point the statistical chance that Janice would survive was still only 25 percent, at best, but the staff did not lose faith, because Janice had youth on her side. The pediatric cases were the ones that could surprise you. Young patients could bounce back unexpectedly from the worst possible situations, ones that always killed adults. Janice had already bounced back twice: from her ambulance ride and from her septic shock. Her youth, innocence, and sweet, unburned face inspired the dedicated staff to see her through, and renewed our motivation to exude a collective confidence that she would make it despite the odds. We were more driven than ever to succeed in our exhausting work.

It can be hard, sometimes, for an ICU staff to keep its spirits up while spending weeks treating a severe sepsis patient. After three or four weeks, as the patient lies there unresponsive and unmoving, the odds of survival fall to extremely low levels. In the case of an adult patient especially, after one month of severe sepsis and unresponsiveness, it is difficult for the staff to keep the faith. After two months the support of these patients can become a chore. After three months there is a danger that the patient will cease to be a real person to the staff. In a sense, a comatose person is by definition devoid of personality. The family brings in pictures of the patient to repersonalize him or her, but if there has been no response from the patient for two or three months, these pictures may not be enough.

There was the case of Mr. Soon, a 56-year-old Korean man who suffered a massive cardiac arrest after an uncomplicated coronary bypass surgery, then developed severe sepsis. I had been assigned to care for him in the cardiac intensive care unit, and for months he lay there, never moving or speaking or responding to me or anyone else. This was in the time before managed care, and hospices. Nowadays the doctors would have the "talk" with the family, explaining that after months of on-and-off battles with severe sepsis, his odds of survival were essentially zero, and that even if he did survive, he would require continuous nursing care and never again live a full life on his own. In today's medical system the family and doctors have come to understand that sometimes the best thing for the patient may be to dial back the treatments, allowing death to come with dignity. Mr. Soon was less fortunate: he was maintained by intensive care for more than a year before he finally died. In many ways he had already been dead to me and the rest of the staff for months.

Modern medicine has accepted a definition of death based on the complete, irreversible loss of brain activity secondary to the death of neurons in the brain. If the brain ceases to function and "dies," then the patient is dead. Severe brain damage does not always cause brain death, however. But it may create situations for chronic care that are extremely difficult for the patient, family, and caregivers. Mr. Soon had suffered severe brain dysfunction from sepsis—he was unable to speak or move—but he was alive. Even today, were I to walk into that cardiac ICU and glance toward the last room on the right, I could conjure up an image of him sitting there, "alive," reclining in his cardiac chair, a white plastic tube connecting his tracheostomy to the respirator, looking at his own swollen legs with blank, expressionless eyes, a stream of spittle running out of the corner of his mouth.

Mercifully, Janice's case of severe sepsis was different, as are most pediatric cases. The youngest ones, especially prepubescent children, can make tremendous recoveries. Janice's staff knew this, stayed strong, and exuded confidence that she would pull through without permanent brain damage. We talked to Janice all the time, stimulating her nervous system, as if she were playing in her crib like a normal child, not allowing ourselves to believe that Janice would die on our watch. She was too loved by her family, and her pretty innocent face held too much promise for a full, rich life.

Death certificates do not typically list severe sepsis as a cause of death, instead assigning causality to clinical conditions that precede severe sepsis, such as cardiopulmonary disease, pneumonia, lung cancer, and complications of a motor vehicle accident. Pathologists dissecting victims of severe sepsis on the autopsy table have revealed some important clues about the syndrome. Like forensic experts at the scene of a homicide, they have scoured the remains of victims, looking for clues or patterns to explain the syndrome's cause. They begin their examinations at the skin and work their way down to the deepest internal organs, collecting tissues along the way that they "fix" by soaking them in formalin. These pieces are later cut into thin sections and studied under the microscope. Autopsy results assign a final diagnosis with profoundly permanent effect. Unlike clinical observations, which evolve and change, autopsy results are the last word in the medical record. The tissue sections can be saved in formalin-filled jars, cataloged in microscopic slides, and stored for decades.

The preserved spinal cord tissues from a paralyzed patient who died 80 years ago, for instance, will still show the distinct, telltale patterns of neuronal death in the motor horns of his spinal cord. These forensic clues are lasting proof that the long-dead patient's disability was the result of polio, because they are the signature of the damage caused by this virus. Compare the pickled spinal cord tissues from a second paralyzed patient. The cells in the cord are normal, but there in the section of the right motor cortex of his brain is clear evidence that some of the neurons that controlled the activity of the arm and leg on the left side of his body were dead before the patient was. Decades after he died, his formalin-fixed brain still reveals that the cause of his paralysis was a stroke, not polio. Even though the yellowed medical records indicate that both victims had muscle weakness in their extremities, the pathology conclusively proves the different causes of their condition.

The pathologist performing an autopsy on a victim of severe sepsis will search for signs of an infection. Sometimes it is obvious, like an abscess in the lung, kidney, brain, or abdomen. But more often than not, a source of infection is never found. Each organ is examined, weighed, handled to assess its texture, then opened up to reveal "gross" changes by visual inspection. It is a time-honored method to diagnose disease after death. Strolling along through an imaginary autopsy gallery of severe sepsis victims, you would be struck not by gross evidence of tissue destruction and death but by the overwhelming normalcy of the organs and their microscopic appearance. Indeed, despite weeks of severe sepsis suffered by the victims in intensive care units, most of these tissues look viable, healthy, and pink. It is difficult to tell which came from the severe sepsis patient and which from the 21-year-old who was in perfect health until minutes before he died of a broken neck from a diving accident. It is uncanny, as if the tissues themselves are begging to ask: Why am I being viewed by you, instead of the other way around?

Very different autopsy results are found in patients who died from acute septic shock. In contrast to the effects of severe sepsis, the residual pathological effects of lethal acute septic shock can be dramatically obvious: blackened fingers and toes; soft, mushy kidneys, adrenal glands, and livers; and extensive tissue damage with inflammation. It is a grossly apparent picture of tissue death and destruction. The episode of septic shock that Janice had endured two weeks earlier had occurred suddenly, coming out of nowhere. The rapidity of acute septic shock and the pathological damage it leaves behind in lethal cases distinguish it from severe sepsis. Severe sepsis tends to progress slowly, spiraling downward on an erosive and destructive course. Janice had survived her septic shock, but if she had died from it, the evidence would have been as obvious as bloody footprints leaving the crime scene. If Janice were to die from severe sepsis, the pathologist would find no such clues.

A recent in-depth autopsy study of severe sepsis victims revealed a dearth of clues indicating the cause of death. The pathologists found some signs of cell death in the spleen and intestines, but what they failed to find was much more significant. Although these patients had died of severe sepsis, there was a paucity of injury or cell death. The pathological changes in the victims were in no way serious enough to account for the overwhelming failure of organ function and patient demise. They wrote: "A fundamental question that remains unresolved despite these extensive histologic studies is the primary mechanism responsible for patient death in sepsis . . . the extent of cell death was not, in general, sufficient to cause organ failure . . . other evidence supports the concept that cell death is not overwhelming in patients with sepsis . . . The absence of histologic evidence of cell death sufficient to explain the morbidity/mortality of sepsis suggests that other, as yet unrecognized mechanisms may be involved in the pathogenesis of the disorder."[17] The implication of these results is that severe sepsis is a different syndrome from acute septic shock.

A number of theories have been suggested to explain how severe sepsis causes widespread organ damage with minimal pathological change. One possibility, proposed by Dr. Mitchell Fink at the University of Pittsburgh, unifies the seemingly disparate complications under one mechanism. He explains: "Patients like Janice, with severe sepsis, develop one complication after the other: renal failure, liver failure with jaundice, pulmonary failure with fluid accumulation in the lungs, and secondary infection caused by bacteria leaking into the bloodstream from the bowels. For the past 30 years we have referred to this as multiple organ failure syndrome, but it is just a name, really, one that belies the fact that we do not understand what is actually going on inside the patient. But the principal organs that fail during sepsis are epithelial organs, meaning that their major functions are dependent upon a layer or layers of epithelial cells that isolate the body's toxins within its organs.

"Epithelial cells form the semipermeable layer between different body compartments, pumping salts, sugars, and proteins from the blood, and then blocking their return. For example, renal epithelial cells prevent urea nitrogen from leaking into the blood, liver epithelial cells prevent bile acids from leaking into the blood, bowel epithelium prevents bacterial toxins from entering the blood, and pulmonary epithelium prevents fluid in the blood from filling up the alveoli. The genius and beauty in the construction of a living organism is that it is divided into carefully controlled compartments, which normal physiology depends on. Failing organs break down their ability to maintain compartments. Epithelial cells form the structural barriers that separate toxins from the blood. If the barriers dissolve, or fail irreversibly, then death is inevitable."

Rather than being tightly connected in an impermeable barrier that prevents toxins from leaking into the bloodstream, in severe sepsis the epithelial barriers fail. A pathologist looking through his microscope would not see any evidence of this; it can only be visualized by means of special staining methods and electron microscopy, which are not used for routine autopsies. It is possible that a drug or device that prevented this type of epithelial leakage would prevent the renal, liver, bowel, and pulmonary failures that kill patients with severe sepsis. In May 1985 we knew that Janice had multiple organ failure and that unless we reversed it she was going to die. We had treated her with powerful antibiotics, and there was no source of bacterial infection. We did not know why her severe sepsis was worsening in the absence of bacteria. So we did the best we could to support her failing organs—to keep her alive—and hoped that the destruction would reverse itself.

six

False Hope

SATURDAY, MAY 25, 1985. After nearly two weeks, Cecilia's prayers were miraculously answered. Janice began to improve. Cecilia said it was a second miracle, the first being her grandchild's recovery from shock. Progress was slow and steady, as if a tape of the onset of her severe sepsis was playing in reverse. Gradually Janice's kidneys and liver began to function again, and the previously leaky epithelial cells began to tighten up and do their job with passing grades—separating the toxins from the nutrients, and cleaning the poisons out of her circulation to restore life to her organs. Once again the endotracheal tube was pulled from between Janice's vocal cords, and once again the respiratory therapist carted the ventilator away. He passed Cecilia at the windowed door, and, recognizing the machine because someone had left a picture of a smiling Janice taped to the side of it, she panicked, assuming that the machine was no longer necessary for the worst possible reason. The therapist, seeing the universal sign of wide-eyed terror on the old woman's face, quickly said that Janice was doing well, breathing on her own, and did not need the respirator any more. With great show and a smile, he peeled the photo off the machine and awarded it to Cecilia as she sobbed. Tears filled his eyes too, and he resumed his walk, pushing the respirator through the door.

We were all thrilled that Janice's luck, and I guess our own, had held, but we did not know what had caused her turn for the better, any more than we knew what had originally caused her turn for the worse. We had sustained her organ function with our infusions and machines, giving them the time they must have needed until they could resume their jobs, and now she had drawn back from the precipice. Dehydrating purgatives and bloodletting had long since been abandoned, so presumably we had not made her worse, but I was not really sure about even that. How could I know if we had made her worse when we did not know what had caused her problem to begin with?

I was relieved for Janice and her family. They smiled now as we discussed this newfound good fortune. But because of my lack of knowledge about the cause of severe sepsis, it did not seem fair to take any credit for treating it. There was no warm glow of self-satisfaction of the kind one feels when prescribing the correct antibiotic to cure a bad case of infection caused by a specific microbe, or successfully removing a diseased appendix. The moment lacked a sense of accomplishment, of knowing that we had found the right answers and done the right things. In reality, we did not know anything then, and we know only a little more now. The two weeks had been like hanging on inside a canoe in white water, fighting forces unseen that tried to dump us into the raging cold water, knowing nothing other than that tomorrow we would be further downstream, condition unknown. I hated not knowing what had happened, and now, 20 years later, I am still looking for explanations. We have some better ideas about severe sepsis now, but the answers are still not all in.

SUNDAY, MAY 26, 12 P.M. Janice was awake and alert, draped over a nurse's shoulder, having assumed the classic baby posture for being burped. She smiled at us when we touched her toes protruding from the dressings on her feet, laughed and wrinkled her nose, and raised her eyebrows to make a funny face. She was cheerful after we removed the nasogastric tube from her nose two hours ago. She finished drinking four ounces of formula from a baby bottle, her first since being burned. The nurse walked in circles next to the crib, gently rubbing Janice's back. The whole scene was starting to look very normal: a small child with a content, post-bottle glow on her face, and a sleepy, comfortable look in her eyes. Her rosy cheeks were evidence of her recovering state; she was healing and regenerating. Her intestines once again processed and absorbed the milk from her bottle, and her brain clearly enjoyed how it tasted and felt. Janice was interacting with her environment. Her brain was responding to her internal and external environments.

TUESDAY, MAY 28. Janice's first birthday party, and everyone was there. They came from the ER and the OR; the respiratory therapists, nutritionists, and renal dialysis nurses; and the nurses and doctors from the burn unit. There was cake and streamers, and the sun was shining. The room was bright and cheery, and Janice was smiling. Her face, untouched by the burning fluid, was not scarred, and it was beautiful. Innocent fun infected the entire burn unit, spread by the smiles on the nurses' faces as they moved down the hall to patients in other rooms. Janice's clear eyes, looking playfully about, beamed when her parents entered the room. Her parents cried tears of joy and hugged their baby and the nurses who loved and cared for her. Cecilia arrived, smiling and murmuring to everyone, "God is good, isn't he? And it's *my* birthday, too! Janice is bet-

ter! What a present, what a gift." There was a great deal to cel-
ebrate, because Janice had beaten the odds and made it. Soon
she would be going home.

Janice had survived the ambulance ride, septic shock, and
severe sepsis. She was eating and gaining weight, and the
steps toward her discharge from the hospital were clear. One
more trip to the OR on Monday, June 3, for relatively minor
surgery to graft a few small areas on the backs of her legs that
hadn't healed, and then home the following week. Her life
would be hard, and she would need splints and therapy for her
arms and legs to prevent the scars from contracting and lock-
ing her joints into a frozen position. She would probably walk
with a limp and have some restricted movements in her fingers, but she would be mobile, and she would probably grow
up to be a fully independent young woman who could even
have children of her own someday. She was going to live. We
shared in that special grace that comes to a winning team of
competent and dedicated individuals. Each knew his or her
own small part in the victory, a contribution dwarfed by the
magnitude of the events. Janice was going home, where she
belonged.

After the party I noticed Maria, Frankie, and Cecilia chatting with the parents of a burn survivor who had come for fol-
low-up treatment at the burn unit's outpatient clinic. The burn
clinic was open every Tuesday and Thursday, from nine to five,
to provide the necessary postburn treatment and wound care to
the burn unit "graduates." Patients had their wounds checked
and dressings changed; plans were formulated for scar excision; and progress was reviewed. A major effort in the postburn period was the prevention of excessive scar formation, for
both cosmetic and functional reasons. Scars can be disfigur-
ing, and they can restrict the range of motion in the joints of
the arms and legs. Postburn care included the applying of

stocking-like nets over burned and grafted sites to reduce scar formation, and the attaching of splints to maintain the functional position of some joints. Aggressive and lengthy physical therapy and rehabilitation was also used to restore and maintain function, a sometimes painful process that could continue for months or years.

Until now Janice's family had avoided the outpatients and their families, even though their waiting spot by the elevators was also the main route into and out of the clinic. During their three weeks of waiting for Janice, they had seen nearly every outpatient come and go. Some were better off than others. The spectrum of residual burn damage and scarring ranged from patients who were wheelchair bound and severely disfigured, to those who appeared completely normal. Secretly they had wondered, like all families of a severely burned patient, where Janice would land on this scale. Today they had begun talking to the parents of a little girl who had survived a house fire. The parents knew all too well what Maria and Frankie were going through because their little girl had been discharged, after a six-week stay in the burn unit, just days before Janice was admitted. I could not hear the discussion, but I could see the body language, and it was clear that the outpatient family had talked about the joy of having their child home again. They exchanged phone numbers, and then, as Maria's and Frankie's eyes brimmed with tears, they hugged and bade farewell to their newfound confidantes.

WEDNESDAY, MAY 29, 1 P.M. It had been a brilliant spring morning, but dark clouds had rolled in from nowhere. There was no rain, but thunder crashed. Janice's room had become shady and dark, like the inside of a cave, with fluorescent light streaming in through the opening facing the hallway. The nurse was feeding Janice a lunchtime bottle, holding her comfortably in a rocking chair adjacent to her crib. Janice was still connected to the cardiac monitor, but other than that the scene looked almost normal, a baby with her bottle, being gently rocked.

As Janice reached the end of the bottle, her eyes suddenly rolled back up into her head, and her heart stopped. The nurse, seeing me walk past the door, called out. I ran in, and seeing a flat line on the cardiac monitor and Janice's face turning blue, I took her into my left arm, covered her nose and mouth with my mouth, and began to puff air into her lungs. I puffed gently, so as not to cause a collapsed lung—a special risk in giving CPR to a small child—and with my right hand, I pressed on her sternum.[18] Gently but firmly, I pushed once every half second, hoping that this external cardiac compression would be enough to keep her blood moving from her lungs to her brain and other organs. About 15 seconds had elapsed from the time her eyes had rolled back until now. I had never given mouth-to-mouth resuscitation to a living person, only to plastic practice dummies in CPR classes, but that did not matter—in my mind I could clearly see everything in slow motion. On my mental checklist, all the boxes were being checked off according to the training I had received. Janice would be fine, I told myself.

I glanced at the nurse and nodded toward the phone, and she called the code. I began to hear the cardiac arrest, or "code," announced on the overhead speakers throughout the hospital hallways. A nameless woman's monotonous voice repeated, "Code red, burn unit," over and over again. Thirty seconds had now elapsed since Janice's heart stopped. I looked up and saw Hal Turnbull jogging through the doorway, a sight I knew assured our success in bringing Janice back because I considered Hal the best surgery resident in the department, an outstanding physician who was training to be a cardiac surgeon and was about to begin his fifth and final year of training. He had received extra training in cardiac emergencies and cardiac procedures, and to me his arrival meant that we would pull Janice through. Hal grabbed an endotracheal tube and laryngoscope from the crash cart that the head nurse had pushed in behind him, and he placed it perfectly on the first try. I connected her tube to oxygen that the nurse had readied, and within three minutes after her heart had stopped, Janice's airway and breathing were secured. Her intravenous catheters were working perfectly, and for the next five minutes we administered drugs according to the cardiac arrest protocol for standstill: atropine, calcium, bicarbonate, epinephrine. Nothing.

The defibrillator was ready. Hal placed the little paddles on Janice's chest, everyone stepped back, and he said "Shock." Her small body twitched all over and we watched the monitor, breathless. Nothing. More CPR, more drugs, and another round of defibrillation. Again, "Shock," but once again no rhythm returned to her heart. This was unheard of! I had been to dozens of codes that were a mess compared with this: when the endotracheal tube didn't go in right, the defibrillator didn't fire, the intravenous lines blew, and the drugs were spilled on the floor. Those patients had all done better than Janice was doing now. What was wrong? More CPR, another round of drugs, and another "Shock." Nothing. The lab results were coming in every five minutes or so, and her blood gases were normal. She was ventilating well through her ET tube and exchanging gases normally. This cycle of CPR, drugs, and defibrillation went on and on, for 85 minutes, as we took turns pushing with our fingertips on her tiny sternum to keep the blood moving through her stopped heart.

At some point in that horrible, shadowy, crowded room, doubt crept in and began to grow. I began to perspire, and I realized that my heart was beginning to race. My mind suddenly lacked clarity; everything was blurry. Something had changed. For the past hour it had not been Janice we were coding; it had been a nameless, faceless individual whose heart had stopped. Now it was all different, as I realized for the first time, *This is Janice we are working on, and we may not get her back!* Today, remembering it all with absolute clarity, I wonder if we had already lost her. The muscles in my chest, arms, and thighs began to quiver, and my knees felt loose, like I was falling.

I was now aware of everything in real time, and it was terrifying. The slow-motion and protective cocoon that had enveloped me during the first hour, when it seemed like I was in control, had dissolved. Now I felt exposed to the pain; I was no longer covered by an insulating layer that slowed everything down and rendered the horrible events into a sterile, intellectual exercise. Reality was fast, racing, and awful.

Janice's heart failed to resume beating, and Hal decided to insert a pacemaker, a sterile wire that could be introduced into the jugular vein and advanced down into her heart. The other end of the wire would be connected to a bedside generator that would produce an electrical current to directly stimulate her heart. I immediately began unwrapping the sterile package and setting out the instruments as he put on his gown and gloves. By now I had ceased working mechanically and felt almost like a spectator at a sporting event where the home team was losing. Alert, anxious, and tremulous, I knew in my heart that this was Janice's last chance. I was also afraid because bedside pacemakers were newly invented for these cases. I had seen them used in a few other codes, but most of the time the device could not be inserted properly, and the results were poor. But I had never been to a code with Hal Turnbull, and miraculously, he positioned the pacemaker into her right atrium on the first try. "This is it," said the little cheerleader in my mind, "just the break we need to turn this mess around. Janice will be fine now."

I turned on the device and watched the cardiac monitor. On cue, the pacemaker began to fire and the electrical signal it generated appeared on the monitor, but there was no heartbeat following it! The heartbeat was not returning. What was wrong?! Every action we had taken in this code had gone by the book and perfectly, but Janice's heart would not beat. We had arrived at the instant she needed us most, and we had breathed for her and pressed on her lifeless chest, but we failed to will her heart back to its rhythmic, contractile purpose. As a medical exercise, the code itself was flawless; its only shortcoming was that it did not bring Janice back to life. She was dead. With life having left her, the microbes could continue their work on her remains.

I did not speak the words; Hal did. "It's over; she's gone." I did not look back, and I never saw Janice again. Exiting her room, I saw to my right the blue-coated gatekeeper, the ward clerk, head down on her desk, sobbing. There were three nurses in yellow paper coveralls standing in the hall; they had come to the code but were not needed and had instead formed a prayer circle, arms around one another's shoulders. Now they held onto one another for support, crying into one another's hugs. I walked into the waiting room, where I delivered the undeliverable news to Janice's mother. Her scream of disbelief and pain is etched into my memory. Even today it summons itself, ghostlike, from some hidden neural sulcus, hurting my heart with a dull ache, and stinging my eyes. Then the newly childless, anguished mother fainted, and I half-carried, half-dragged her to the pink-plastic-lined waiting room couch, where I positioned her limp head on the lap of her own sobbing, incoherent mother, Cecilia, who had spilled the boiling water. Then I went to the nursing station to fill out the paper-work and sign the death certificate.

I could not talk about Janice's case with anyone for months, and I developed recurring dreams of her failed code. Unlike the real event, in which my brain had given me some protection and distance from the tragedy of her death, in these dreams I was completely unprotected—I experienced each of them with anxiety, frustration, and terror. Most telling, from the outset of every dream I knew she would die. I frequently awakened yelling orders for drugs or saying "Shock," perspiring, breathing fast, and feeling both sad and angry. Since that time I have spoken to countless physicians and nurses about their memories of patients whom they lost. The pediatric cases leave the deepest scars.

Dr. Brett Giroir, the pediatric intensivist, noted that codes in children are inevitably unforgettable: "The memories of a pediatric cardiac arrest are surprisingly visual and graphic, starting with the mass difference between the 15 or 20 adult doctors and nurses all surrounding and working on a 22-pound kid. That's a ratio of 3,000 pounds to 22 pounds! And at the time it is all happening like a slow-motion video; you are in a different zone, where there is no thought of individuals or time or space."

I told Brett about Janice, and he immediately recalled his "Janice": "I remember in 1983 there was Brittany, a little 4-year-old who was fine when she went to bed at night, but awoke in the morning with a fever and a rapidly progressive rash. A meningitis outbreak had been in the news, and her mother, fearing the worst, raced her to our hospital. Along the way the girl, becoming stuporous, said, 'Mommy, don't worry about me, I'm going to be in heaven today.' She arrested as soon as she arrived in the intensive care unit. Even by today's standards she had outstanding medical care; the right antibiotics, the right steroids, the right intravenous fluids, and all the right monitoring devices. There were at least four ICU attendings, God knows how many fellows and nurses, and we worked on her for four or five hours. But it did not matter; it was done. Game over. Her death particularly affected me. I felt forced to seek new treatments, look for other therapies, because I could not tolerate not being able to do anything to stop the disaster. At least not while I just stood around and waited to see if it would happen again the same way.

"Everything could even go perfectly by our medical standards," he said, after a moment, "but for some diseases it doesn't mean that you can do a damn thing to stop it from happening. One thing that you never get used to, even if you see it lots of times, is a child's funeral. I hate little coffins. There is something wrong with a little coffin; they are not meant to be three feet long. Coffins are meant to be eight feet long. A three-foot coffin means 50, 60, or 80 years of unfulfilled promises. You can't live your life as a physician accepting that you can't do something about it. Her death directly affected me; it influenced all my professional choices for 20 years."

I never saw Cecilia or any of Janice's family again, and I do not know what happened to them after that day in the hospital waiting room. I have often wondered about Cecilia and what could have happened to her. Did she go on? If so, how? The scalding was an accident, but Cecilia must have felt responsible. She spilled the boiling water in a scene that I have imagined hundreds of times when turning to my own sink, carrying boiling water, thinking to myself, "Where is the baby? Are all the kids away from my feet?" How many times was that scene replayed in Cecilia's mind? And did it always look the same?

C. G. Jung described the case of a woman who during a therapy session confessed to having "murdered" her daughter.[19] Jung discovered this by performing association tests, during which she elaborated the details. She had been home and depressed, and while bathing her child gave her a glass of river water. The woman knew that the river water in her area was never to be used for drinking because it was tainted with typhoid and other lethal, disease-causing agents. Soon after, the child died of typhoid fever. Before her therapy with Jung, she had completely denied the event, even to herself, and her depression severely worsened. She was institutionalized soon thereafter.

Jung wrote: "I told her everything I had learned [about the child's death] through the association test. It can easily be imagined how difficult it was for me to do this. To accuse a person point-blank of murder is no small matter. And it was tragic for the patient to have to listen to it and accept it. But the result was that in two weeks it was possible to discharge her . . . she departed bearing her heavy burden. She had to bear this burden . . ." Perhaps Cecilia sought therapy from a psychologist, psychiatrist, or her priest, and maybe they helped her find the inner strength to bear her heavy burden.

Another possibility, suggested by Dr. John Kane, executive director of the Zucker Hillside Hospital in Queens, New York, is that Cecilia's ability to survive this psychological assault is somewhat analogous to surviving an infection. Just as the immune response can be beneficial and appropriate, or excessive and inappropriate, so too can be the emotional or psychological response to causing an accidental death. Dr. Kane explained: "The event, in this case the accidental scalding of your own granddaughter, is like the pathogen. The person's response is dependent upon her personality, her genome, her experiences, and her own level of development of successful and beneficial adaptive responses to stress. But like the immune system, which can be responsible for a range of responses that span the entire spectrum from insufficient to beneficial to excessive to harmful, the individual's response to a stressful or catastrophic event can be insufficient, appropriate, or excessive. With a healthy or adaptive response, the memory of the event recedes with time. It is tempered, and, while not forgotten, it is moved back to a safe distance from day-to-day activities and life. Thinking about the event elicits an appropriate level of sadness or sorrow that does not interfere with the individual's ability to live and to function.

"If the person has an insufficient adaptive response, then the memory does not recede. Minor events like the sound of a baby laughing or crying, or the smell of pasta cooking, trigger an active replay of the scalding. A vivid memory occupies center stage, a reenactment of the entire scene, over and over, in a paralyzing manner that is incompatible with normal life. These individuals are at risk for post-traumatic stress disorder. At the other extreme are people who have an excessive adaptive response. They suppress the event to the point that they deny that it ever occurred. This denial is also unhealthy; it will cause significant distress later. The key to a successful resolution of these tragic events is a balanced adaptive response."

TUESDAY, JUNE 18. I received a manila envelope in the mail containing the report of Janice's autopsy. We were required by law to refer her case to the New York Medical Examiner for an autopsy because she had died after an accidental burn. I had hoped that the report would contain answers to the major question of her case: Why did she die? Unfortunately, it contained no answers. Instead, it noted in simple, dry pathological prose that her organs "appeared normal, there was no evidence of significant tissue damage, inflammation, pulmonary embolism, heart disease, or infection." The cause of death was listed as "cardiopulmonary arrest," a phrase I knew the office had merely lifted from what I had written as the cause of death on her death certificate. They found nothing wrong, nothing to explain why she died. Twenty years later, I have some theories but still do not know with certainty.

seven

Unraveling Shock

My mother died when I was 5 years old. I do not remember much about her short illness, caused by a brain tumor, but I do remember talking to her father soon after the funeral. My grandfather, Charles Culotta, was a pediatrician, and a professor of pediatrics at Yale, where for many years he had performed scientific research on the causes of infectious diseases, including whooping cough and polio. In 1939 he published one of his papers in *Science*, a study of the transmissibility of polio via public sewage. After my mother's funeral we were talking in the office he kept in his home, a small, crowded room tucked behind the dining room. He sat in his favorite chair at the desk, and I climbed up onto his lap—breathing deeply the cigar smells that were richly absorbed into the green leather chair and that permeated the books lining the walls from floor to ceiling.

I asked him why the neurosurgeon hadn't simply removed the brain tumor so that my mother could have come home to us. He patiently explained the problem—one that is still unsolved today—that this type of brain tumor (a glioblastoma multiforme) had spread its tentacles deep into otherwise normal regions of her brain. It would have been impossible to remove those tentacles without severely damaging or even removing large parts of her normal working brain. This would have ruined her life. I decided then that I wanted to do research someday, to try to discover ways to reduce the suffering caused by disease. I wished to prevent some other child from experiencing the sadness I felt. My grandfather pronounced that a fine plan, then reached across his desk and handed me a precious memento—a squirrel monkey skull that he had used for his polio research. It was about the size of a tennis ball, mounted on a small, thin piece of mahogany, and he always kept it on the corner of his desk. As I write today at my own desk, it is there looking at me as it used to look at him.

Twenty-two years later, in July 1985, I had finished two years of training as a surgeon, and Janice was gone. I was about to begin a two-year stint of scientific research, doing experiments and writing papers. During this time I would not be caring for patients or doing surgery; afterward, I would return to the hospital and complete my training as a neurosurgeon. It was time for me to pick a research project, and I was having nightmares about Janice, haunted by the mysteries of her battles against septic shock and severe sepsis. What had happened to her? What had caused it all? Were there really any "circulating toxins"? And couldn't we make an antidote rather than waiting around for complications to develop? I started down a scientific path looking for answers to these questions, and I am still following it today.

I began doing research in the laboratory of Steven Lowry, a surgeon at Cornell University Medical College renowned for his expertise in the metabolic responses to injury. We collaborated with a prominent scientist, Anthony Cerami, who was then dean and head of a large laboratory at Rockefeller University. For several years Cerami had been trying to find the cause of the debilitating weight loss that complicates chronic illness. Cerami discovered that this lethal wasting syndrome, termed cachexia, was caused by a protein made by the immune system. At first the identity of the protein was unknown, but it later became clear that it was a cytokine, one of the proteins produced by immune cells to coordinate the response to infection and injury. Cerami and Bruce Beutler isolated the protein, naming it cachectin for its activity in causing cachexia.

Amazingly, at about the same time, this protein was discovered independently by Lloyd Old at Memorial Sloan-Kettering Cancer Center, directly across the street from both Rockefeller University and New York Hospital's burn unit, on New York's Upper East Side. Old had been studying proteins released by macrophages in their battle against tumors, so he named the protein tumor necrosis factor, or TNF, the name the cytokine is known by today. We now understand a great deal more about TNF's role as a member of the cytokine family. Like other cytokines, TNF is produced by the immune system to perform a number of tasks, including cell-to-cell signaling that coordinates the activities necessary to defend the host against a bacterial assault. When white blood cells encounter bacteria, they respond by producing a variety of cytokines, including TNF, and releasing them into the infected area. This sends clear messages that "bacteria are not welcome here" and "the immune system is activated to fight." Cytokines are a mainstay in the immune system's arsenal.

At the time that I began working in Steve Lowry's laboratory, Cerami and Beutler had just published a tantalizing paper in Science. They said that blocking the activity of TNF in mice conferred a small but significant protection against the lethal effects of a bacterial toxin. It seemed possible, therefore, that TNF might be dangerous not only to the bacteria but also to the host. I wondered if this presumed defender might actually be the "blood poison" that caused Janice's acute septic shock. Theoretically, even a small number of bacteria, too few to detect or find in a given patient, might be enough to trigger a burst of TNF sufficient to activate a lethal sequence of shock and tissue injury. The sudden release of TNF, rather than the bacteria, might be the cause of rapidly progressive shock and organ damage.

To study this possibility, I set up a "rodent intensive care unit" on the sixth floor of Cornell University Medical College, in the laboratory of Dr. G. Tom Shires, chairman of the Department of Surgery, who supported my efforts in these early years. Working on an anesthetized rat, I exposed the carotid artery with microsurgical instruments and created an opening in the side of the vessel two tenths of an inch wide. I threaded a small, fluid-filled tube through this tiny hole and connected the other end to a pressure transducer, a device that would measure the blood pressure inside the artery. Each heartbeat now produced a pressure wave that was measured on a video screen and printed on a paper chart, a re-creation of the monitors on the wall next to Janice's crib. It was absolutely essential to begin with studies of septic shock in rodents, not test tubes: there was simply no other way to sort out this complex problem involving living, functioning physiological systems.[20]

Working in Cerami's lab at Rockefeller, Beutler exhaustively produced and purified large amounts of TNF, which I carried across the campus to my rodent ICU at Cornell and infused into the intravenous catheter of the anesthetized rat. The results were startling: within minutes, its blood pressure fell and the rat went into profound shock. The heart rate increased at first, as the rat's nervous system and circulatory system worked to try to compensate for the diminished blood pressure. This failed, however, and the rat's blood pressure continued to fall. As in Janice's shock, the rat's arteries had dilated, causing the blood pressure to plummet. Its respiratory rate tripled, a response that we later learned was due to a massive buildup of lactic acid in the bloodstream. The lactic acid had lowered the blood pH from a normal of 7.4 to 6.9, a level of acidosis incompatible with life. Acidosis in this range triggers the brain to increase the respiratory rate in an effort to expel more carbon dioxide and raise the blood pH to normal levels. Blood sugar levels increased at first, but soon they also fell, to levels low enough to impair brain function.

Then, suddenly, the rat died. Its blood pressure fell to zero, and it stopped breathing. I quickly split open its chest and observed that the heart was still beating—but there was no strength or efficiency to the contractions, the arteries had become lax, and there was no blood pressure. Five minutes later, supported neither by blood pressure nor by respirations, the heart finally stopped beating. The similarities to Janice's case of shock were astounding—the onset of shock had been sudden and devastating—and in both cases no bacteria were implicated in the process. The conclusion was inescapable: all you needed to develop acute shock like Janice's was too much TNF.

At first it was difficult to believe. TNF, a protein produced by normal macrophages in every man, woman, and child, could be a lethal molecular weapon that caused shock. I repeated this experiment dozens of times and the results were always the same: exposure to high levels of TNF caused lethal shock and tissue injury, with severe, widespread damage in the lungs, kidneys, and intestines. Under the microscope it was clear that the blood vessels had become clogged with white blood cells. It looked as if the presence of TNF had activated every white blood cell in the body, turning them into uncontrolled, roving gangs of street fighters. Their rush to battle was like a stampede, as they crushed themselves into the smaller blood vessels, blocking all movement of the blood downstream.

These clots of white blood cells diminished delivery of oxygen-carrying blood to the tissues, creating ugly purple "ischemic" lesions that marked zones of cell death. TNF made the blood vessels sticky, causing clots to adhere to the walls of the small arteries, which blocked the flow of blood. Large sections of the rat's bowel were ischemic, and in places the cells lining the bowel wall itself were dead, suffocated by a shortage of blood. As the cells lining the bowel wall died, the protective barrier between the bacteria-filled bowel contents and the bloodstream was eliminated, enabling bacteria and toxins from stool to enter the bloodstream. It was striking that the immune system itself produced the death factor that caused acute shock. The body's front line of defense against microbes, the police force designed to protect and to serve, was capable of killing the patient. And it could do so very quickly.

JULY 1985 THROUGH SEPTEMBER 1986. I studied these shock-inducing effects of TNF for more than a year, repeatedly observing that it caused falling blood pressure and widespread organ damage. I presented my findings at a weekly Monday morning laboratory meeting, which was a forum to discuss new research results and to generate feedback from the senior scientists and physicians in attendance. Afterward, a prominent surgeon-scientist raised his hand and commented, saying simply, "You must be wrong; it can't be true. Why on earth would the immune system make a protein that kills the patient?" The explanation then, as now, lies in the *amount* of TNF produced. Low-level production of TNF is a crucial part of the normal immune response—it facilitates the killing of bacteria, the remodeling and healing of injured tissues, and the activating of long-term immune responses that can protect against subsequent infections. These and other activities of TNF are clearly beneficial. As long as the amount of TNF produced is regulated, and held within the nontoxic range, the patient benefits, but if TNF is overproduced, it is toxic.

This wouldn't be the first discovery that a "normal" biological substance could be dangerous when overproduced. Medicine is rife with examples of damage caused by the uncontrolled release of normal hormones, too. Some tumors are like uncontrolled hormone-secreting factories, producing insulin, epinephrine, or antidiuretic hormone; the hormone levels rise to extremely high levels that in turn cause specific and potentially life-threatening side effects. In some cases a lethal tumor can be as small as 5 mm across and nearly impossible for a surgeon to find. The tumor itself does not directly kill the patient, however; it kills precisely because it has become an unregulated hormone-manufacturing site releasing excessive, toxic amounts of molecules that would normally benefit the patient when produced under tight control. We also knew that allergic reactions—like those caused by a bee sting, for instance—can lead to an overproduction of histamine by mast cells. Low levels of histamine are important to host defense, but the sudden release of large amounts, as occurs when the victim is allergic to bees, causes shock and respiratory failure. Before the discovery that TNF itself caused shock, septic shock had not been seen that way—shock was not considered a problem of immunological excess. The idea that it might be such a problem prompted a great deal of controversy.

OCTOBER 1986. We published the shock-inducing effects of TNF in *Science*, and the article elicited widespread interest. We received dozens of letters and phone calls from scientists and investigators around the world who wanted to participate in the research. Many people, like the senior surgeon at the lab meeting, doubted that the immune system played a causative role in acute shock. As happens in medicine and science, time has diluted the surprise of this discovery. The shock-inducing and proinflammatory activities of TNF are now accepted dogma, taught in medical school lectures and described in the standard immunology, medicine, and surgery textbooks. The lethal side of TNF is now known to be part and parcel of its amino acid sequence and protein structure. But in those early days, the idea of a "bad acting" component to TNF or any other immunological molecule was viewed with considerable skepticism. Some denounced the theory as improbable at best; to others it was simple heresy. The controversy subsided only after many laboratories had replicated the results, establishing without doubt the potentially dangerous side of TNF.

I focused next on the practical issues inherent in developing a new treatment, wondering whether it might now be possible to spare shock victims like Janice from the potentially lethal consequences of excessive TNF. In the autumn of 1986 we started the critical experiments necessary to apply this concept to patients. We first developed an antidote against TNF—a molecule, termed an anti-TNF monoclonal antibody, that specifically bound to TNF, neutralizing its toxicity. We proved that the antibody effectively prevented the action of TNF in cell culture experiments. Then we were ready to test the antidote by administering the antibodies to primates with a real bacterial infection. For this purpose we developed an animal model of septic shock in baboons, an abundant, nonendangered primate species that is anatomically and physiologically similar to humans.

Two anesthetized baboons lay on their backs, side by side on adjacent operating tables in a large animal operating facility designed for experimentation on the eighth floor of the Cornell University Medical School. We performed surgery to place catheters into the femoral arteries and veins in the baboons' groins, and connected the arterial line to cardiovascular monitors that were functionally identical to those used in intensive care units. We threaded catheters through the baboons' femoral veins all the way to the heart, following the course of venous blood through the right atrium, right ventricle, and out into the pulmonary artery in the lungs. A balloon at the end of the pulmonary catheter could be inflated intermittently to measure the "pulmonary artery wedge pressure," an indicator of blood volume and cardiac function. For this experiment to be successful, it was critically important for us to control all of these parameters, treating the baboons just the way we treated our patients in the burn unit's intensive care beds, on the seventh floor of the adjacent hospital building, less than 1,000 feet away.

The microbes we selected for this study were a strain of bacteria originally isolated from a patient with septic shock. We knew that injecting the bacteria intravenously would cause the baboons to develop septic shock. In this way we could study whether the baboons made TNF before they developed septic shock, and, most important, whether we could prevent the condition using the anti-TNF antibodies. We knew that TNF, while a crucial component of the immune response, could be toxic, but we did not know what would happen if we blocked it with the antibodies. One possibility was that blocking TNF, this major weapon in the immune response to infection, would cripple the baboons' immune systems, freeing the bacteria to proliferate wildly, and making things far worse instead of better.

The major difference between these baboon studies and the earlier rat experiments was that we administered live bacteria, which caused an infection in the bloodstream. These microbes would stimulate the baboons' own immune systems to make TNF, rather than us giving the animals TNF that we had made in the lab. We treated one of the infected baboons with the anti-

TNF, which specifically inactivated the baboon's TNF by binding to it, covering it up, and rendering it essentially invisible to the baboon's tissues. The other baboon received an irrelevant antibody that did not bind to TNF. For the next eight hours we treated both baboons with intravenous fluids. We increased or decreased the intravenous infusion rates guided by a treatment protocol, based on blood pressure and urine output, identical to that used in hospital intensive care units.

The differences between the baboons' responses were as startling as they were profound. In both animals the bloodstream TNF levels increased significantly and rapidly, beginning minutes after the bacteria infusion and reaching peak levels within two hours. The unprotected animal developed shock, and within six hours it stopped producing urine. In the eighth hour it died. The other baboon, which had been treated with anti-TNF antibodies, was completely protected from shock. It remained stable, with normal blood pressure, heart rate, and respiratory rate, and its kidneys and other organs continued to function even after the untreated animal was dead. Although both baboons had received identical bacterial infections, only the recipient of the anti-TNF was protected against the development of shock. Our conclusion was striking and immediate: TNF, not the bacteria, caused lethal septic shock.

Two years after Janice's battle, we had discovered that TNF was the cause of septic shock. TNF, not the bacteria per se, was the source of the "blood poisoning," or "humoral imbalance," that underlies it. This experiment had clearly demonstrated that the syndrome of septic shock could be dissociated from the presence of the bacteria. The bacteria are not directly responsible: rather, macrophages and other immune cells responding to the bacteria produce TNF, which in turn causes shock and tissue injury. Our findings explained why Janice had developed septic shock even though we had not found any microbes: her immune system had produced too much TNF.

This was an incredible "eureka" moment, one of those elusive and memorable events that occurs, at best, only occasionally in a scientific career. Scientists and medical researchers can doggedly pursue the answer to one question for years, poring over thousands of experimental results yet never finding the answer they seek. Thomas Edison said, "The first requisite for success is the ability to apply your physical and mental energies to one problem incessantly without growing weary." Driven by a need to know, most scientists define their own existence by the problems they have solved and the answers they have provided in their papers, patents, and lectures.

Research is difficult, in part because there is intense competition for money, lab space, and supplies. Today's successful scientists direct large teams of people, driven to pursue their individual experiments. They go to work to slay mythical dragons, along the way becoming nearly immune to the pressures created by experimental failures, rejection of their new ideas by their colleagues, and loss of research funding. These drawbacks may temporarily deter them, but they persist, flitting from idea to experiment to the results and back again, hoping that years of work and searching will produce the answer to the "big question." If that day comes, it can come suddenly and unexpectedly.

If the scientist happens to find herself alone at the eureka moment, she is likely to become frenetic, looking for someone to tell. This scenario can prompt (later infamous) phone calls to distant colleagues in the middle of the night. Discoverers have been known to run down to the basement to grab a janitor or night watchman, anyone who happens to be in the building, to come to the lab and share in the moment. "Just look through this microscope, Bill, see how different the left is from the right! I found it! I found it!" Bill looks, then returns to his work, cleaning the floors or guarding the front door. He smiles not at the left-right difference, which meant absolutely nothing to him, but at the gleeful transformation he saw on the face of the scientist. The discovery altered the discoverer, a person who had seemed lost in thought for years, who rarely made eye contact with anyone and who never smiled, until just now.

Six of us were together the night of the baboon experiment, so I did not have to go running around the building to share the moment. My colleagues Tony Cerami, Steve Lowry, Yuman Fong, Kirk Manogue, and David Hesse and I stood around the veterinary operating tables until 3 a.m., discussing the impact that this new concept could have on medicine, and wondering about the potential implications for human health. At dawn the antibody-treated animal showed no sign of shock or tissue injury, so we removed the catheters and returned it to its cage. It awoke from anesthesia without any obvious side effects, and within 24 hours resumed eating, moving about, and living normally, fully alive.

In December 1987 we published these results in *Nature*, in an article demonstrating for the first time that monoclonal antibodies against TNF could be used as an experimental drug. The broad implication of this discovery was that the immune response to an infection had the potential to cause tremendous harm. Our observations flew in the face of a major, time-honored premise in the field of immunology: that immune responses are, almost by definition, beneficial to the host. The stage was set for testing anti-TNF monoclonal antibodies in patients, an approach that would lead to a new class of drugs now widely used to improve the lives of patients with diseases caused by excessive TNF release.

In 1987 it became clear to us that TNF was both necessary and sufficient to cause an acute shock syndrome during infections, but unfortunately, our results also indicated that it would be impractical, if not impossible, to use antibodies to treat septic shock in patients like Janice. The problem was that to protect the baboons completely, the antibodies had to be onboard *before* TNF levels increased and triggered shock. TNF is produced so suddenly in cases of septic shock, and acts so quickly to cause tissue injury, that antibodies would have to be given either before bacteria appeared on the scene, or within the first few minutes afterward. Without a medical crystal ball to predict future episodes of infection or septic shock in our patients, we were stymied in our ability to treat patients like Janice, because their TNF peak would occur without warning. It was not going to be possible to treat most victims of septic shock before its onset, and giving anti-TNF antibodies would not undo the damage once TNF had started the sequence of shock and tissue injury.

Janice had survived her battle against septic shock. If she had succumbed to it, however, her autopsy would have revealed a distinct pattern of tissue injury from TNF poisoning: blackened organs, and small hemorrhages covering her skin with a rash composed of rose-colored rings. This is a pathological picture similar in many ways to the septicemic plague, though the plague is rarely seen today. A more common form of TNF-mediated septic shock occurs during infection with the bacterium *Neisseria meningitidis* (meningococcus). Lethal outbreaks can occur in epidemics, like one that killed 16,000 people in West Africa in 1996. Meningococcal infection of the bloodstream (fulminant meningococcemia) causes a highly lethal, rapidly progressing acute syndrome of septic shock, with fever, plummeting blood pressure, a spreading reddish rash, purple hemorrhages into the skin, and blackened limbs. It kills up to 15 percent of patients, often in 24 to 48 hours. Autopsy of these victims reveals inflammation in the skin and heart; inflamed blood vessels, termed disseminated vasculitis; irreversible damage to the adrenal glands, termed adrenal necrosis; as well as acute damage in other organs. These pathological changes closely resemble those in TNF-poisoned animals. Patients with fulminant meningococcemia have developed some of the highest TNF levels ever reported in humans, comparable to the levels we observed in animals with acute shock caused by TNF toxicity.

Today I understand that Janice's acute septic shock, like shock during fulminant meningococcemia and probably acute septicemic plague, was caused when the immune system suddenly overproduced TNF and released it into the bloodstream. Septic shock caused by excessive TNF is a distinct clinical-pathological syndrome that occurs in some, but not all, patients who develop an infection. Sometimes, as in fulminant meningococcemia, a previously healthy individual can suddenly develop acute septic shock. In other cases, like Janice, an injury or surgery can render the patient more vulnerable to an overproduction of TNF. Common precipitating causes occur in patients hospitalized after surgery for trauma, cancer, or other diseases. Pneumonia, appendicitis, and infections in other organs can predispose patients to the development of septic shock, in each case because the immune system becomes overstimulated to the point that its weapons, such as TNF, cause damage to the patient as well as to the bacteria.

The discovery that TNF causes shock was translated, relatively quickly, to the clinic, a huge undertaking that would not have been possible without the historical background research upon which the treatment of infectious diseases is based. Louis Pasteur formulated the germ theory of disease in 1864, suggesting that living microorganisms cause infectious diseases. This principle focused scientific research on bacteria instead of the humoral imbalances theorized by Galen centuries before. Pasteur implicated microbes rather than humors after discovering that microbial life was necessary for fermentation, a process that had previously been attributed solely to chemical reactions, not microorganisms. Pasteur proved that microscopic bacteria or yeast carried in the air could contaminate a brewing mixture, causing a healthy solution to become "diseased" and ferment. He developed methods to prevent fermentation by either killing the microbes or blocking their access into the liquids. Pasteur also built his theory on observations he made while searching for a method to remedy a silkworm disease that was crippling the French silk industry. He noticed that healthy silkworms became ill after they resided on the same leaf as diseased worms, and realized the disease was caused by transmission of microbial pathogens. Pasteur's germ theory has dominated infectious-disease research for more than a century.

One of the earliest practical applications of the germ theory to human disease was developed by the British surgeon Joseph Lister, who introduced "antisepsis" in 1867. After reading Pasteur's work, he reasoned that microbes might be involved in the development of postoperative infections. To kill the microorganisms, he applied a spray of carbolic acid, a widely used sewer cleaner, to his surgical instruments, postoperative wounds, and bandages, a process later dubbed Listerization. His approach significantly reduced the mortality from infection after limb amputation and other surgeries. This was a major revolution in thinking about the role of microbes in human disease, and it spawned a durable quest for the Holy Grail of infectious-disease research: a method to eradicate the lethality of infection by killing pathogenic microbes. Adoption of sweeping public health and sanitation measures reduced the transmission of pathogenic microbes through drinking water, the air, and human touch. The widespread eradication of so-called transmission vectors, such as the rats and fleas that carry plague, significantly reduced the mortality attributable to infectious diseases in the overall population. Mortality declined even before the production in the twentieth century of antibiotics for clinical use.

The development of effective infectious-disease treatments that specifically targeted individual bacteria came to rely on a theoretical framework for assigning blame for a specific disease to a particular microbe. This framework or paradigm,[21] from which nearly all subsequent therapies for infectious diseases have been derived, was proposed by the German physician Robert Koch. Koch worked out a method for isolating cultures of pure microbes by applying diluted mixtures of bacteria onto a culture medium composed of gelatin, or agar. This enabled the isolation of individual bacterial colonies derived from a single ancestor cell, free of contaminating microorganisms. Armed with the ability to identify specific organisms, in 1884 Koch developed the basic rules or "postulates" that bear his name and that revolutionized research on the treatment of infectious diseases. Researchers still use these rules to determine whether a causal relationship exists between an agent and a specific illness.

In summary, Koch's postulates require that the agent is found in every case of the disease; the agent can be isolated and cultured; inoculating the agent into a naive live animal causes the disease; and the agent can then be recovered from that animal. When an organism or agent fulfills Koch's postulates, it is said to be a necessary and sufficient causative agent for the disease. Koch applied his postulates to studies of several infectious diseases, including anthrax and tuberculosis, proving that the individual agents were both necessary and sufficient to cause disease. Koch received the Nobel Prize in physiology or medicine for his work, and more than a century after his death, the principles he developed are still assiduously applied to identify the cause of newly emerging infectious diseases—for example, SARS.

Pasteur and Koch (along with Edward Jenner, Ilya Ilyich Mechnikov, and others) have been included among the founding fathers of the field of immunology, the science of the cells, molecules, and organs that provide immunity against infections and invasion. The word *immunity* comes from the Latin root *immunis* meaning "free of"; the term originally referred to being free of taxes but was adapted to mean free of disease. On July 6, 1885, Pasteur injected his rabies vaccine into 9-year-old Joseph Meister, whose parents had brought him to Pasteur. They were certain that the child had received his death sentence two days earlier, when he had been bitten by a rabid dog. Rabies at that time was 100 percent fatal. Pasteur had developed a weakened, or "attenuated," rabies virus, which he hoped would not cause a severe form of rabies but would still be capable of activating the immune system to attack it. He isolated a rabies virus from a fox, then weakened it by growing the virus in rabbits. He was then able to recover a strain of the virus from the rabbits, which he administered to the boy. Meister lived, becoming the first documented human rabies survivor in history, and within a few years Pasteur's therapy was used successfully in thousands of cases. Despite the success of the vaccine, the science of immunology had no explanation for how it actually worked.

In 1883, Ilya Ilyich Mechnikov suggested that specialized cells provide a layer of defense against bacteria. His theory emerged from his studies of motile cells in starfish larvae. When he introduced small foreign objects (tiny thorns from a tangerine tree) into the larvae, he saw that they became surrounded by specialized, mobile cells. These cells ingested the thorns, leading him to wonder whether a similar process might occur in more complex animals. He deduced that white blood cells could perform this function of a front-line defense by entering sites of infection and inflammation, where they could ingest microbes. The consumption of foreign objects and bacteria by white blood cells was termed phagocytosis, and mobile white blood cells capable of performing this process were named phagocytes. This work led to the theory of cellular immunity, for which Mechnikov received the Nobel Prize in 1908.

Mechnikov shared the Nobel Prize with Paul Ehrlich, a proponent of the theory of humoral immunity, which proposed that the major immune defense against infection was not the white blood cells but noncellular "humoral substances" that circulated in the blood. These substances included antibodies that traveled in the circulation, where they could bind to and neutralize toxins. Today we understand that cytokines in the bloodstream are another important component of the humoral response, but Ehrlich's studies were focused on antibodies, or "antitoxins." The method he developed to standardize the activity of any antiserum is still used today to test antibodies before their use in the clinic.

The cellularists, led by Mechnikov and his phagocyte theory, and the humoralists, led by Ehrlich and his antibody theory, fought for prominence. This intellectual battle lasted through the first half of the twentieth century, with each side arguing that its theory was the dominant basis for all immunity and that the other theory was a minor component. For 50 years the humoralists won out and the major focus of immunity research was on the protective actions of antibodies, and other components of humoral immunity that kill bacteria and neutralize toxins. Today, however, immunology recognizes the importance of both cellular and humoral immunity in the defense against bacterial infection.

In the late twentieth century, medicine capitalized directly on the therapeutic power of individual antibodies. Georges Köhler and César Milstein invented a method to produce identical antibodies against a specific target or antigen. Before, it had only been possible to collect pools of diverse antibodies from the circulation of animals or humans inoculated with an antigen. These "antiserums" contained a mixture of many hundreds or thousands of differing antibodies that could be difficult to separate, purify, and standardize. Köhler and Milstein solved this problem by developing a method to produce identically cloned cells, each constituting a single antibody. They did so by fusing an antibody-producing cell with a tumor cell. All of the progeny of this cell produced an identical antibody, termed monoclonal. This revolutionized medicine, which had previously relied on polyclonal antibodies from serum as the basis for many diagnostic tests and treatments. The development of monoclonal antibodies made it possible to mass-produce identical antibodies for use in patients. Köhler and Milstein's work earned them the Nobel Prize in 1984.

Not until the 1980s did it become clear that molecular messengers produced by the immune system, such as cytokines, could actually cause disease, or that monoclonal antibodies that block the molecules could be used as a therapy. This work led ultimately to what I now refer to as the cytokine theory of disease, which proposes that molecules the immune system produces can cause disease. According to this revolutionary theory, passive immunization against a specific cytokine (such as TNF) could in theory effectively prevent specific disease manifestations. Suddenly the focus shifted from developing treatments based solely on eradicating an infectious agent to targeting products of the immune system. Decades of experience with antibiotics had made it abundantly clear that some patients died even though the germs causing their illness were killed and all traces of microbial pathogens eradicated. Antibiotics reduced the mortality of bacterial infections, but alone they did not guarantee that infected patients would live. Now we knew, for cases of septic shock at least, that if the immune system released too much TNF, shock and tissue injury could progress regardless of the bacteria's fate.

Although Koch used his postulates as the basis for identifying the causative role of a pathogenic microbe that can reproduce itself, we can consider the shock-inducing action of TNF under a similar light. TNF is present in cases of septic shock, and it can be isolated from animals and humans with the disease. Inoculating TNF in healthy animals reproduces the disease in a naive host, and although TNF cannot reproduce itself like a microorganism, it can be recovered from an animal with shock caused by exposure to TNF. Finally, animals that cannot produce TNF are protected against the development of acute septic shock. TNF is thus a necessary and sufficient causative agent of the disease. Acute shock can occur whether bacteria are present or not because TNF, not bacteria, causes the disease.

In the late 1980s the technology for creating and mass-producing monoclonal antibodies had advanced to the stage at which it was possible to safely produce large quantities of highly specific anti-TNF monoclonal antibodies for human clinical trials. This was a period of tremendous excitement, and several biotechnology and pharmaceutical companies established large development programs based on the concept of using anti-TNF monoclonal antibodies as a drug. Business and sales models were uniformly optimistic in predicting that the first drug proven to effectively prevent infectious-disease deaths would be a billion-dollar blockbuster. Tens of millions of dollars were allocated for production and testing, creating significant industrial pressure to produce and develop monoclonal anti-TNF for use in severe infection.

Separately, Marc Feldmann and Sir Ravinder Maini of Imperial College, London, discovered a role for TNF in rheumatoid arthritis, a debilitating autoimmune disease of the joints that causes pain, stiffness, warmth, redness, and swelling. Painful inflammation in the "synovial" tissues lining the joints primarily in the wrists, fingers, elbows, and knees destroys the adjacent cartilage and bones, causing gross deformity, misalignment, and ultimately immobility. Two million people suffer from rheumatoid arthritis in the United States today, and many of them are disabled by the disease. The cause of rheumatoid arthritis is still unknown, so treatments are based on blocking inflammation by a combined use of corticosteroids, nonsteroidal anti-inflammatory agents such as ibuprofen and aspirin, and other drugs (for example, methotrexate, leflunomide, D-penicillamine, sulfasalazine, and gold-containing compounds). Despite treatment with these drug cocktails, many patients fail to receive effective relief.

Feldmann and Maini found that inflamed synovial tissues and joint fluid of rheumatoid arthritis patients contained high levels of TNF. They theorized that perhaps the proinflammatory activity of this cytokine could stimulate downstream tissue damage in the joint, triggering a destructive inflammatory response, similar to the manner in which TNF stimulates tissue injury in distant organs when released systemically. To determine whether the inflammatory activities of TNF contributed to joint destruction in arthritis, they administered anti-TNF antibodies to animals with experimentally induced arthritis and observed that the treatment conferred significant protection against the development of painful, red, and inflamed joints. Centocor Inc. was in the advanced stages of producing an anti-TNF monoclonal antibody for human clinical trials; Feldmann and Maini persuaded the company to use it in a clinical trial of rheumatoid arthritis patients.

They realized almost immediately that anti-TNF was a powerful treatment for these patients. In Feldmann's words: "What the patients noticed first was relief from fatigue. Their mood improved, and by the next day, the pain and stiffness had lessened and they were feeling remarkably better. And this benefit continued for a period of weeks, so in this initial trial there was virtually instant evidence suggestive of clinical benefit."[22] Larger trials soon proved the therapeutic efficacy of anti-TNF antibodies, now known as Remicaide. It and similar drugs have received approval in the United States and other nations for the treatment of rheumatoid arthritis. Feldmann and Maini received the prestigious Albert Lasker Award for Clinical Medical Research in 2003 for their important work.

These successful results with anti-TNF validated the cytokine theory of disease in humans and changed medical practice. Millions of anti-TNF doses have been administered, and although it is not effective in all patients, it has proved to be the most significant therapeutic advance for rheumatoid arthritis in decades. Children with juvenile rheumatoid arthritis, who previously suffered from serious complications of corticosteroid treatment, including stunted growth and weight gain, have been restored to normal activity levels at home and school. Youngsters whose growth had been severely stunted from regular steroid use prior to the availability of anti-TNF have now returned to normal on their height and weight charts. Anti-TNF therapy has been approved for the treatment of Crohn's disease, another autoimmune disease, affecting the bowel. TNF inhibitors already provide billions of dollars in sales revenue to the pharmaceutical industry for arthritis and Crohn's disease, and further uses for other diseases are likely.

Janice's story presaged much of the early work on TNF in acute septic shock, as well as the later development of TNF-inhibitor therapy for rheumatoid arthritis, but unfortunately, the efforts to develop a treatment for acute septic shock based on the cytokine theory of disease were decidedly less cheery. To understand what happened, it is important to reiterate that septic shock, like the case Janice had during her first week in the burn unit, is an acute syndrome defined by falling blood pressure and other signs of infection. It comes on suddenly, occasionally in previously healthy individuals, but more frequently in patients, like Janice, who are already injured or sick. Untreated septic shock can be rapidly fatal, sometimes within hours, and it leaves distinct pathological evidence of tissue damage and cell death. Severe sepsis is a distinctly different syndrome that should not have been lumped under the same diagnostic rubric as acute septic shock. A large body of preclinical work had defined TNF as a drug to treat septic shock, not prolonged or severe sepsis. Severe sepsis is a protracted illness that comes on slowly and leaves little or no pathological evidence in its wake.

If the term severe sepsis seems to describe something bewilderingly complex, do not despair. You are not missing something, and you are in good company. Numerous international scientific conferences during the past 25 years have focused widespread attention on the definitions of sepsis, and the magnitude of the unresolved problem. Participants are scientific and medical experts in critical care medicine, the specialists who care for patients with severe sepsis. The definitions have been molded and crafted by passionate debate and lively discussion about including or excluding particular signs and symptoms. The clinical criteria necessary to diagnose severe sepsis have been revisited and rehashed time and time again. As noted earlier, patients receive a diagnosis of sepsis if they have developed combined abnormalities of body temperature, heart rate, respiratory rate, or white blood cell count. They are diagnosed with severe sepsis when they have these signs of sepsis in addition to organ damage in the lungs, liver, cardiovascular system, kidneys, or brain. Patients diagnosed with severe sepsis can actually have one of many different underlying diseases that trigger it; it is not a single entity. While it may be convenient for some purposes to lump patients together under a name, as for instance to calculate allocation of intensive care unit resources necessary for these critically ill patients, it was an inelegant and inexact approach for enrolling patients into a clinical trial for anti-TNF.

However, semi-blinded by optimism bordering on euphoria about blockbuster new drugs, clinical researchers in the late 1980s readily speculated that anti-TNF would provide the first major new approach to treating infectious disease since antibiotics. Market forecasters projected that sales revenue from a drug used to treat anyone with "sepsis" would amount to billions of dollars annually. This excitement created tremendous pressure on business leaders to fund a trial that might capture the entire market by being first in the sepsis race. The quarry: a modern-day "magic bullet" 100 years after Paul Ehrlich had coined the term—one drug to fit anyone lying in an ICU bed. This flawed approach took our early studies of animals with shock out of context, and, despite advice to the contrary from us and others, several companies launched clinical trials to demonstrate that anti-TNF could be used to treat patients with "sepsis," not just "septic shock." Decision makers ignored the differences between septic shock and severe sepsis and launched trials that enrolled patients with severe sepsis, whether they had shock or not.

This strategy might have been reasonable if most or all patients with severe sepsis went on to develop acute shock, but that is not the case: only a small fraction of severe sepsis patients develop acute septic shock. As a result, thousands of patients with severe sepsis were enrolled in trials of anti-TNF that cost tens of millions of dollars to complete; the vast majority of these patients did not have septic shock, the disease on which the antibodies had originally been used in animals. While organizing and implementing these huge clinical trials was difficult and expensive, the expectations remained high, so when the results came in showing that lives were not saved, the failure sent shock waves of negative news and disappointment rippling through the headlines in both the scientific and medical journals, as well as on the business pages. What went wrong? What had been overlooked? A lot.

First and foremost, several advisers had pointed out before the trials that the design basically violated Koch's postulates. Our early work in animals, which had since been independently confirmed by many others, had established that TNF is a causative mediator of septic shock, not severe sepsis. Virtually all of the major preclinical work using monoclonal anti-TNF was performed in animal models of a distinct syndrome of septic shock: lethal tissue injury with discrete pathological changes in specific tissues, and serum TNF at extremely high levels. This model was characterized by a rapidly progressive syndrome quite similar to Janice's sudden shock, and quite distinct from sepsis. Not only did the vast majority of patients who received anti-TNF in clinical trials for sepsis not have septic shock but, perhaps worse, with few exceptions they did not even have any detectable TNF levels in their serum.

Moreover, in the few patients who did have detectable TNF, the serum levels were orders of magnitude less than those that caused shock in animal models. After the trials had begun, and thousands of patients had been treated, independent scientists began to report that anti-TNF antibodies were not effective in animal models of sepsis without shock. Anti-TNF antibodies not only failed to protect animals from lethal experimental peritonitis without septic shock, in some experiments the anti-bodies actually *made the animals worse.* The distressing result of these studies was that TNF did not fulfill Koch's postulates as a causative agent of sepsis without shock in animals.

There were more problems. The trials used patient inclusion criteria painted with the widest possible brush strokes, to include anyone with severe sepsis. Patients young and old, with cancer, gunshot wounds, and pneumonia, were lumped together in these trials in a large, heterogeneous group labeled severe sepsis. This approach was unprecedented in modern medicine. Consider, for example, the treatment of cancer, in which a powerful, highly effective drug for leukemia is quite useless against a tumor in the colon. Each of these diseases is indeed "cancer," but effective treatment depends on additional information about the underlying processes that drive individual types of disease. Unlike Feldmann and Maini's discrete approach in patients with confirmed rheumatoid arthritis, whereby they first obtained solid evidence in animal models that TNF fulfills Koch's postulates, the anti-TNF sepsis trials were initiated without comparable results that TNF was a necessary and sufficient mediator of sepsis without shock.

A justifiably worrisome extension of the anti-TNF sepsis trials was that inhibition of normal TNF levels in a simmering infection might actually worsen the outcome. Theoretically, blocking TNF at nontoxic levels could actually reduce the immune system's effectiveness in protecting against infection, giving an advantage to the germs and allowing their uncontrolled proliferation. Years later this proved to be exactly the case, and there have been some cases of patients who received anti-TNF antibodies whose underlying infection worsened. Low levels of TNF are indeed protective against some types of infection, so anti-TNF antibodies are usually discontinued if an infection develops.

The report of failed trials was disturbing to many but came as little surprise to the advisers who had earlier urged a more cautious, restricted approach to the clinical trial design. An effective trial would have included patients with shock who were more physiologically, pathologically, and immunologically similar to the animals we had studied. One reason for resistance to this more selective approach was that it would have been prohibitively expensive. It would also have been difficult to identify patients with acute septic shock early enough in their disease course to enable timely intervention with anti-TNF. It is true that the ideal study would have been extremely difficult to implement, and would probably have taken several years longer to complete, but at least it would have provided a scientifically meaningful answer. The original preclinical animal results using monoclonal anti-TNF in baboons in 1987 indicated that the best time to treat with monoclonal anti-TNF was *before* the onset of maximal TNF levels. A next-best scenario would be to treat patients early during TNF-mediated shock, as occurs during acute bacterial meningitis and in some cases of bacterial infection after trauma or pneumonia. Treatment would begin at the earliest signs of shock, or perhaps in people at the highest risk of developing it: patients like Janice who had severe burn injury, or those with sudden-onset meningococcal infection. It is theoretically possible that inhibiting the extremely high levels of TNF in these patients might reduce the progression of organ damage and improve the chances of recovering from shock.

To me there was another tragedy of this flawed clinical trial of sepsis without shock: more than 20 years after I treated Janice, I still do not know whether anti-TNF therapy might be an effective treatment for patients with acute septic shock caused by excessive TNF. Today, some of the investigators who participated in the anti-TNF sepsis trials believe that their patients who were in shock actually received some benefit from monoclonal anti-TNF. These results exist primarily in the form of anecdotes that merely tease the imagination but cannot render a valid, statistically supported conclusion. These "clinical observations" linger in the air, wafting about as untested possibilities and unrealized hopes that perhaps a patient with acute septic shock lying in an ICU near you might derive some benefit from anti-TNF. A clinical trial designed to treat patients in septic shock or at high risk of septic shock, modeled after our early studies in baboons, is still needed. It is possible, indeed likely, that some patients with acute septic shock have a syndrome caused by TNF, as we have been reviewing here, but this does not exclude another possibility. It is theoretically possible that there are other, as yet unidentified, mediators that also cause acute shock and tissue injury, independent of TNF; anti-TNF antibodies would not be effective for this other type of syndrome.

eight

Unraveling Sepsis

The effectiveness of anti-TNF in rheumatoid arthritis patients proved that a drug designed to target a specific
causative component according to the cytokine theory of
disease can effectively treat the disease. Now, ten years after the failed anti-TNF sepsis trials, there is only one FDA-
approved drug for severe sepsis, and it is only effective in
a small percentage of patients. As far back as the fourteenth century, physicians distinguished between the
acute septicemic and the more chronic bubonic forms of
the plague. I hope that future trials will not lump together
diverse patients with different infections at widely different points in the progression of their disparate diseases.
One may justifiably wonder whether biotechnology has
raced ahead of our ability to test products in people with
severe sepsis. I do not think so. Instead, I believe that the
approach of the clinical trials of the past decade simply
diverged far from the parsimony of Koch's postulates.

The answers are not in, but I envision that future trials will enroll patients, and controls, based on clinical
criteria, standardized disease duration, genomic data
about cytokine and cytokine receptor expression, and direct molecular evidence that the target mediator is pres-

ent and active in a specific patient. Only when a specific treatment is analyzed in patients who have the specific target molecule will it be possible to determine whether our pharmaceuticals of the twenty-first century will improve survival from our modern pestilence.

JULY 1994. Nine years after Janice's hospitalization, we still did not understand the cause of severe sepsis. I was convinced that the presence of bacteria alone could not provide all the answers because, as in Janice's case, microbes are not always present. In 1993, working in my Laboratory of Biomedical Science in the Department of Surgery at North Shore University Hospital, in Manhasset, Long Island, I introduced an alternative approach to the problem of severe sepsis based on the hypothesis that a previously unrecognized mediator might be responsible. The immune system makes hundreds of cytokines, and I decided to search for one that might cause severe sepsis. I began by reasoning that the putative cytokine, if it existed at all, would not be produced until a considerable time after the onset of infection. This thinking was based on the fact that severe sepsis is a slowly progressing disease; it also carried the implicit hope that if such a delayed molecule was indeed responsible, then it might be possible to intervene with monoclonal antibodies before all the damage was done.

We distilled this complex problem down to an issue of timing, suspecting that if there were a cytokine (or collection of cytokines) that caused a slowly progressive syndrome like severe sepsis, its release would coincide with the development of the signs and symptoms of the disease. One relatively common cause of severe sepsis is peritonitis, an intra-abdominal infection caused by spillage of bowel contents after perforation, as in the case of a perforated appendix or ulcer. This disease can be experimentally introduced in animals by surgically creating a bowel perforation; this causes a lethal disease that progresses slowly, over three to seven days, like severe sepsis. Peritonitis in animals and humans causes death a relatively long time after the infection. At the time of death, animals, like humans with sepsis, have relatively nontoxic amounts of TNF in their blood—not the high levels associated with shock, as noted earlier.

The physiological and pathological findings after lethal peritonitis are very similar to those found in severe sepsis: diffuse organ injury in the kidneys, liver, and lungs, but without microscopic evidence of tissue inflammation or "necrosis," a process that causes cellular components to become swollen and rupture. Peritonitis causes a slow, prolonged activation of the immune system, with increased cytokine release that can persist for days. The trick would be to find a cytokine that appeared at the time severe sepsis developed, and to block its activity so as to prevent the development of lethal organ failure such as we had seen in Janice.

Ona Bloom joined my lab fresh from Barnard College in New York. Confident and enthusiastic, she could be found at her bench in the lab every morning at 6:30 a.m., despite her protests that she was "not a morning person." Ona began studying macrophages, looking to see whether they released a cytokine as a delayed response to infection. She focused her efforts on the proteins released 18 or more hours after the macrophages became activated by exposure to bacterial products. After months of work she isolated a candidate protein that fit the bill, but it was an inauspicious start—we were extremely disappointed when its amino acid fingerprint identified it not as a cytokine but as a protein known as high mobility group B1, or HMGB1, a constituent of the nucleus of virtually all living cells.[23] This was decidedly not the hoped-for eureka moment. We concluded that the project had been a complete bust and that our discovery of HMGB1 was an artifact of our cell culture conditions, caused by the death of a few cells that had released their HMGB1 when they died. Frustrated and disappointed at our bad luck, we conceded that HMGB1 was not the cytokine mediator of severe sepsis.

We were downtrodden primarily because HMGB1 was a well-known protein that was a critical component of normal cells, one of the most abundant molecules in the cell nucleus, and a regulator of DNA structure and function, having nothing to do with a battle fought by the immune system. The principal functions of HMGB1 were to facilitate gene transcription and stabilize complex DNA structures. It seemed that we had isolated not an immunological factor, or therapeutic target for severe sepsis, but an experimental accident. We put this project behind us and moved our attention elsewhere.

OCTOBER 1994. Months passed with little thought or word of HMGB1 in the lab meetings or discussions. We continued to study cytokines and severe sepsis and to read the scientific literature in these areas, and only occasionally would HMGB1 crop up. In the back of my mind, however, I was nagged by the thought that maybe HMGB1 really *was* a mediator. The idea simmered and stewed, and then slowly, and surprisingly, the more we looked at it, the more it seemed possible that HMGB1 could be fit into a cytokine pattern. We began to put together a "what if" scenario, constructing a theory of how one might possibly envision HMGB1 as a cytokine. What emerged was extremely interesting.

The work of Heiki Raulvala's laboratory in Finland indicated that HMGB1 could be found on the surface of particular cells: namely, the brain cells called neurons. The research suggested that this "cell surface form" of HMGB1 functioned like the rudder on a ship, steering growing neurons to make contact with other neurons. This was intriguing because we knew that many cytokines, including TNF, can be found on the surfaces of macrophages before being released into the extracellular space. Could this additional role in neurons be a clue that HMGB1 was not simply a nuclear protein that we had accidentally purified from the macrophages? That maybe it really was a cytokine released by macrophages when they became aroused or activated? Perhaps HMGB1 had a second job, working outside the cell as a cytokine when it was not busy performing its better-known "normal" job in maintaining DNA structure and guiding the growth of neurons.

JULY 1995. Ona Bloom left my laboratory to earn her doctoral degree at Rockefeller University, and the HMGB1 project was picked up by Haichao Wang, a research scientist with outstanding expertise in molecular and cell biology. Haichao is a thoughtful and talented scientist who revels in working on hard, high-risk projects. He had been working at the University of North Carolina in Chapel Hill, but we persuaded him to move to New York despite the fact that while he was being interviewed for the job, the air bag was stolen from his rental car. Living on a postdoc's salary, he could ill afford the insurance company's deductible payments, and I feared that in annoyance he would return to Chapel Hill as quickly as possible. The lab administrator, Dee Prieto, saved the day, however, and hooked the recruit by kindly explaining that this one bad day was atypical and that he should not be deterred from the excitement and thrills of New York. Fortunately, he decided to come and take on the HMGB1 project.

For nearly two years Haichao worked diligently, cloning the gene that produces HMGB1, perfecting the purification methods necessary to make large quantities of protein, and finally inoculating the protein into rabbits to produce antibodies.

Then he used these materials as molecular tools to measure the levels of HMGB1 in the serum of severe sepsis patients. The levels were much higher than we had considered possible, and that the highest levels were present in the serum of the patients who had died. Comparable HMGB1 levels were also found in mice exposed to lethal doses of bacterial endotoxin (a toxin of internal origin), and once again the highest levels were measured in the mice that died. Like the results in the macrophages, the increased HMGB1 levels in the mouse serum occurred only after a delay of 12 to 18 hours from when the mice were exposed to endotoxin. The evidence all pointed to the possibility that HMGB1 was produced as a later-arriving mediator, or facilitator, in a time frame that suggested it might be involved in the development of severe sepsis.

Haichao then developed anti-HMGB1 antibodies as a therapy for use in situations in which HMGB1 was overproduced, including lethal endotoxemia. The antibodies he produced neutralized HMGB1, but not TNF, and they completely protected mice against the lethality of endotoxin. Haichao observed major differences in the appearance of treated and untreated animals and could tell just from looking at them whether they had been treated with anti-HMGB1. Antibody-treated animals were more alert and active and exhibited normal feeding and grooming behavior, whereas the untreated, control animals were significantly less active, moved slowly, avoided feeding, and instead huddled in the corners of their cages. As a final proof of the role of HMGB1 in these mice, Haichao found that administering purified HMGB1 to normal animals caused a lethal syndrome of organ dysfunction, but not shock.

JULY 1999. We published these findings in *Science*, in a paper that demonstrated that HMGB1 can function as a delayed cytokine mediator of lethality. This study provoked a tremendous amount of interest in the biology of HMGB1 as a cytokine. In a collaboration with Ulf Andersson, a pediatric rheumatologist and professor at the Karolinska Institute in Stockholm, we published in the *Journal of Experimental Medicine* in 2000 the discovery that HMGB1 can activate macrophages to produce TNF and other cytokines. The results were clear: HMGB1 was both a nuclear protein and a cytokine. When released outside the cell, it was capable of causing death and activating an immune response. Five years after we thought our search had ended in failure, we redoubled our efforts to study the role of HMGB1 in animals with peritonitis, to see if it was responsible for causing severe sepsis.

Huan Yang, a fiercely competitive and intellectual experimentalist who had joined my lab in 1999, found that septic mice developed extremely high serum levels of HMGB1, but only after the now-expected lag period of 18 to 24 hours from the onset of peritonitis. HMGB1 levels remained high for days, coinciding with the period of severe sepsis. Huan then administered HMGB1 to mice and examined whether the toxicity of HMGB1 in normal animals caused a pattern of injury that resembled severe sepsis. Careful study of HMGB1-poisoned animals revealed that they developed neither shock nor gross tissue injury. When examined after death, their organs appeared uniformly well preserved, without obvious evidence of necrosis, tissue damage, or hemorrhage; except for small inflammatory lesions in the liver, and minor ischemic changes in the heart, the tissues appeared normal at the microscopic level as well. These findings were comparable to the changes seen in patients who died of severe sepsis. Mice exposed to HMGB1 developed other signs of a "sickness syndrome," including fever, decreased activity, withdrawal, increased sleeping, food avoidance and anorexia, decreased pain thresholds, and loss of sexual activity. It therefore appeared that HMGB1 itself could cause a lethal disease that was similar to severe sepsis.

Finally, Huan studied the effects of anti-HMGB1 antibodies in mice with lethal peritonitis. Animals that received an irrelevant "control" antibody, which did not neutralize HMGB1, remained severely ill and lethargic and huddled together in the corners of their cages, avoiding even food and water. This was in stark contrast to the animals treated with anti-HMGB1: within hours of receiving the antibody, their activity had increased, and they resumed eating, drinking, and grooming themselves normally. The anti-HMGB1 had restored or rescued the animals from near death: 80 percent of the control animals died, compared with only 20 percent of the animals treated with anti-HMGB1. The anti-HMGB1 antibody was quite specific—it did not interfere with TNF or other known cytokines—yet it had significantly blocked the progression to death in mice with severe sepsis.

FEBRUARY 2004. These results, which established that HMGB1 is a causative agent of severe sepsis in mice, were published in the *Proceedings of the National Academy of Sciences*. At the time of this writing, efforts continue toward completing the work necessary to possibly translate this idea into a drug. There are a number of advantages to using antibodies to prevent the toxicity of cytokines, a major one being that antibodies used as drugs are extremely specific, meaning that they interact only with one specific target, in this case HMGB1. We have observed comparable protection from lethal severe sepsis with the use of a nonspecific experimental drug that prevents HMGB1 from being released. My colleague Luis Ulloa treated mice with ethyl pyruvate, a widely used food preservative discovered by Dr. Fink (chairman of the critical care medicine department at Pittsburgh) to have anti-inflammatory properties. The mice had significantly lower serum levels of HMGB1 during severe sepsis, and were also protected against lethality. The paper that we published, also in the *Proceedings of the National*

Academy of Sciences, demonstrated that these independent strategies to block HMGB1 significantly reduced the lethality of severe sepsis. Together with the other evidence, it is clear that HMGB1 is a necessary and sufficient mediator of lethal sepsis in animals.

We had yet to find out how HMGB1 actually caused the clinical signs of the syndrome and the characteristic organ damage. Dr. Fink and his colleagues discovered that HMGB1 caused epithelial dysfunction similar to that in patients with severe sepsis. When HMGB1 was applied directly to epithelial cells, they became leaky, losing their ability to function as a barrier. The HMGB1 did not cause the cells to separate from each other, but it did cause the connections between the cells, which normally form a tight barrier, to dissolve. This change occurred at the molecular level; it would not be observable by the standard microscopic methods typically used during the autopsy of a victim of severe sepsis. These results allowed us to formulate a unifying explanation for the way in which high levels of HMGB1 during severe sepsis cause organ dysfunction: HMGB1 makes the epithelial barrier leaky, which in turn allows metabolic toxins to find their way into the bloodstream. It is quite possible that the leak-causing effects of HMGB1 could also contribute to the leakage of fluid out of blood vessels, which, as we saw in Janice's case, is a major problem that leads to dehydration and necessitates the infusion of large amounts of intravenous fluids. This theory explained not only the clinical signs of epithelial organ failure and the buildup of waste products in the bloodstream during severe sepsis but also the autopsy results.

During infection, HMGB1, like other cytokines, is released when bacterial toxins or cytokines, such as TNF, activate macrophages or other responding cells, including neutrophils, endothelial cells, and epithelial cells. This explains the high levels of HMGB1 in patients with infection, but what about the patients who are not infected but have severe sepsis? Where does their HMGB1 come from? For this theory to be complete, it should also offer a plausible explanation for this other facet of the puzzle. Importantly, the HMGB1 theory of sepsis provides such an explanation: injured and dying cells can release HMGB1 from the large reservoirs normally found inside living cells. Injury or ischemia can cause cells to die by "necrosis," a process that causes cellular components to become swollen and rupture, releasing the large quantities of HMGB1 normally stored inside cellular compartments. This simple explanation has significant implications for patients with severe sepsis, many of whom, like Janice, do not have evidence of active microbial infection, but do have extensive tissue damage, which itself can be a source of HMGB1. Janice's burn wounds could have released HMGB1. Other tissue injuries, broken bones, and hemorrhagic shock can also lead to cell damage and HMGB1 release. Once released, the HMGB1 can cause epithelial barrier failure and organ dysfunction, a process that would be clinically indistinguishable from the development of severe sepsis as a complication of bacterial infection.

I do not mean to imply that HMGB1 is the only active mediator in the complex processes that make up severe sepsis. It surely does not act alone. But it appears to occupy a pivotal role that serves to bridge the clinical observations of patients who have infections and those who do not. HMGB1 released from either the immune system or cell necrosis activates the immune system to produce dozens of other cytokines, including the classical proinflammatory cytokine mediators. The mixture of these cytokines increases or decreases the direct activities of HMGB1 itself. For instance, small amounts of TNF cause a highly significant increase in the actions of HMGB1, amplifying the potential for toxicity and tissue injury. And HMGB1 can influence the activity of other cytokines that contribute to the progression of organ damage. Although this theory can explain a great deal about what is happening to cause organ damage in animals with severe sepsis, the caveat is that animals' immune systems differ from those of humans, and thus their response to severe sepsis may have major differences as well. We can cure severe sepsis in laboratory animals, and, as of this writing, only hope for a similar result in patients.

What has emerged from the discovery that HMGB1 acts as a cytokine is a possible explanation for the puzzle of severe sepsis. Unless problems arise, such as unanticipated toxicity from anti-HMGB1 antibodies, it is possible that some clinical trials will begin soon. The HMGB1 cytokine theory continues to gain acceptance, as more data and clinical observations come in, but the final determination will come from trials in humans.

Evolution clearly did not maintain HMGB1 as a major structural component throughout the vertebrate animal kingdom just to provide scientists with an opportunity to come up with a new theory of severe sepsis. Since multicellular organisms first appeared on the planet, they could be killed by infection or injury. The viability of a species depends on its capacity to mount protective responses, activate defensive measures directed against pathogens, and mobilize energy stores to support protein synthesis and other requirements for repairing the damage from injury or infection. Evolution likely capitalized on HMGB1 as a mediator because it would not normally be released; it would be released only if the cell had become damaged or leaky.

A high level of HMGB1 floating in the extracellular space is a signal that damage has occurred. As it travels away from the site of cell damage, HMGB1, like a weather service emergency alert system, notifies other cells that a problem has occurred. Large amounts of HMGB1 are normally locked safely inside the cellular compartments, so if it escapes, then other cells know that something has gone wrong somewhere in the organism. It is a kind of molecular alarm that "something is rotten in the state of Denmark." Another benefit to releasing HMGB1 is that in some cases it can kill bacteria directly. This antibacterial action of HMGB1 fits nicely into our theoretical scenario, in which an infection causes a cell to die, which in turn releases HMGB1. This cytokine then travels in the extracellular milieu and bloodstream, fulfilling two distinct functions: it is an internal, ready-to-use, primitive antibiotic, dispensed as needed, and a molecular alarm signal. Evolutionary parsimony uses HMGB1, like other cytokines, to multitask. This works fine when low, beneficial levels of HMGB1 are produced; problems arise only when large amounts are released.

The pathological mediator role of extracellular HMGB1 is not restricted to the problem of severe sepsis, because HMGB1, like TNF, can also cause arthritis. HMGB1 released into the joint space causes the development and progression of inflammation and arthritis. Ulf Andersson and his colleagues made the crucial discovery that the inflamed joints of patients with arthritis contain high levels of HMGB1. They observed similar results in mice subjected to experimental arthritis, indicating that HMGB1 is found in association with the disease in humans and animals. When they injected HMGB1 directly into the joint space of a mouse, it caused a robust inflammatory response, and clinical signs of arthritis. The administration of anti-HMGB1 antibodies to mice with experimental arthritis ameliorated the disease. So it appears that HMGB1, like TNF, is a causative mediator of arthritis in mice. The inciting events of rheumatoid arthritis are not known, but I believe that once inflammation begins, the resultant cell damage and macrophage activation in the joint cause further release of HMGB1, which in turn worsens the tissue damage. Anti-HMGB1 antibodies interrupt this cycle in animals, and attenuate the damage. They may be effective in humans too, but clinical trials have not yet been performed.

This newly developed knowledge about the mediator role of HMGB1 came years after Janice's battle against severe sepsis, so we cannot prove that HMGB1 caused her disease. I suspect that it did, however, and that HMGB1 also contributed to the bubonic form of the fourteenth-century pestilence, the syndrome that killed slowly without shock. In the future it may become possible to identify specific individuals in whom HMGB1 plays a causative role in severe sepsis. As I've mentioned, HMGB1 may not be the causative agent in *all* patients with severe sepsis, and clinical signs alone may not distinguish these patients from each other, so it will be important to determine which patients with severe sepsis actually have an HMGB1 type of the disease. The task before us is clear: learn how to target future therapies to specifically address the causative agent in an individual patient. This may prove to be a difficult undertaking, but it is not without precedent. Today doctors already expend tremendous effort to isolate and identify specific pathogenic bacteria in critically ill patients. This information is used to guide the prescription of antibiotics to the individual patient from whom a specific organism is found. I believe that in the future, doctors will focus significant effort on identifying not just the microbes, but the cytokine or cytokines that cause specific diseases in individual patients. This information will be used to prescribe specific treatments.

Preclinical work is proceeding as necessary to implement clinical trials of anti-HMGB1 antibodies. It is possible that the antibodies may cause some unanticipated side effect, though we have not observed any in our animal studies. They may block a normally beneficial role of the protein, but this seems unlikely because anti-HMGB1 antibodies do not interfere with the normal function of HMGB1 inside the cell, and it should be possible to treat only patients that have abnormally high, dangerous levels of HMGB1 outside the cell, as occurs in sepsis and arthritis. I believe that one day it will be possible to diagnose and treat severe sepsis not only by describing the organs that fail, an activity that we have in common with our fourteenth-century physician predecessors, but also by therapeutically targeting HMGB1, or another to-be-discovered cytokine that causes the disease in a particular patient. Alas, there may not be one magic bullet for all who come to the ICU, but targeted approaches based on specific causative cytokines such as HMGB1, or other molecular agents, may yet prove effective.

nine

Brain Control of the Fatal Sequence

The discoveries that TNF overproduction can cause septic shock, and that HMGB1 overproduction can cause severe sepsis, suggested two significant questions: Why does this cytokine overproduction happen in some patients but not others? And how is the release of TNF and HMGB1 normally controlled, so that the decidedly unhappy events of cytokine excess are prevented? Recent discoveries about the nature of these cytokine-controlling mechanisms, and how they work, have yielded important clues about how to prevent excessive inflammation. It now seems possible that Janice's septic shock and severe sepsis occurred because of a breakdown or malfunction in the neural pathways that normally suppress or restrain cytokine release. Amazingly, the nervous system, under the direct control of the brain, normally provides the brake on the immune system: your brain can prevent the fatal sequences activated by excessive TNF or HMGB1. The consequences of a failure in this system are dire, like brake failure in a fully loaded truck rocketing down a twisting mountain road.

The good news is that your brain, as your command-and-control center, precisely regulates the amounts of TNF and HMGB1 produced during an injury or invasion. The central nervous system continuously receives incoming data about the status of the immune system, getting its news from the front as messages in nerve fibers. After processing the information, it sends orders back to the front, directing the battle. Commonplace wounds and low-level infections with viruses or bacteria activate the immune system to begin producing cytokines, but the brain monitors the quantities of cytokines produced. If the levels become dangerous, the brain can activate protective mechanisms to halt further cytokine release. The result is a highly coordinated and amazingly effective self-defense network that protects you from yourself. It keeps you safe so that you do not lapse into septic shock or severe sepsis every time you get an infected pimple, hangnail, or scratch from your faithful cat.

MANHASSET, LONG ISLAND, AUGUST 1993. This relatively new knowledge about the neural control of cytokine production came serendipitously. Progress in science is often made by surprise, when an observation from one experiment answers another question entirely. A revelation of this sort occurred in my lab at North Shore University Hospital (the lab is now part of the Institute for Medical Research). It led us to discover that the nervous system controls the immune system's release of cytokines. Marina Bianchi, a creative and enthusiastic graduate student known for constantly scribbling notes to herself on her palms with a blue pen, had been working on a chemical method to switch off TNF production in macrophages. She was studying a molecule that we had developed and named CNI-1493, when she noticed that it blocked the production of TNF and other cytokines made by cultured macrophages. This immediately suggested that it might be possible to use CNI-1493 as an experimental anti-inflammatory agent to prevent the overproduction of TNF.

For five years we pursued the possible uses of CNI-1493 in animal models of inflammation, arthritis, shock, sepsis, infection, stroke, brain injury, and inflammatory bowel disease. On the surface these diseases (and their animal models) are dissimilar, but closer inspection reveals that an overproduction of TNF plays a role in all of them. Treating the animals with CNI-1493 suppressed TNF synthesis and significantly improved the outcome from each of these diseases. This led us to publish a series of papers defining the anti-inflammatory potential of this molecule. By the time these preclinical studies were completed, I was convinced that CNI-1493 acted directly on a fundamental regulatory control point governing the ability of the immune system to produce TNF, but we had no idea how.

The "accident" occurred as we studied the effects of this molecule in rats with experimental stroke. Stroke is brain damage caused when blood flow to a region of the brain is blocked, creating a condition termed cerebral ischemia. Blood-deprived neurons begin to die from a shortage of oxygen and glucose, normally carried into the brain by the bloodstream. The problem is compounded, however, because the cells in the zone of ischemia begin to overproduce TNF. The overproduction of this cytokine makes matters significantly worse for the neurons that are struggling to survive; it adds to the brain damage, killing some cells already suffering from the shortage of oxygen and glucose. We had already showed that administering anti-TNF antibodies lessened the extent of brain damage, and we now decided to use CNI-1493 to block TNF synthesis in animals with stroke. We were not surprised that CNI-1493 significantly inhibited TNF production in the brain and reduced the damaging effects of stroke. We were also not surprised that injecting CNI-1493 directly into the brain was more effective than giving it intravenously, because more drug was available in the ischemic brain region when we placed it there directly than when it arrived via the bloodstream.

We were surprised one day when the experiment was done wrong; the results unleashed a series of subsequent experiments that culminated in an amazing find. The mistake occurred when CNI-1493 was injected into the brains of rats as part of a study of endotoxemia, not stroke. Endotoxemia causes extremely high, shock-inducing levels of TNF to accumulate in the bloodstream. When the results came back, we were incredulous to find that the presence of extremely low doses of CNI-1493 in the brain completely blocked the synthesis of TNF in the bloodstream. This was wholly unexpected, and difficult to explain, because the doses of CNI-1493 in the brain were well below the quantities necessary to block TNF production in the entire immune system. Yet somehow it had happened, and CNI-1493 in the brain was 300,000 times more effective than CNI-1493 in the bloodstream. Astonishingly, it appeared that the brain had somehow "sensed" or detected the presence of CNI-1493 and responded by signaling the immune system to stop producing TNF! It seemed that somehow the brain had usurped the entire immune system by overruling the authority of the macrophages on the front line—commanding and controlling a complete shutdown of cytokine synthesis.

The implications were striking, intriguing, and important; this finding suggested that we now held the key to understanding a major regulatory or controlling point that could inhibit TNF synthesis throughout the entire body. At the same time, it made teleological sense, because clearly there would be a benefit to the host if the brain could prevent the immune system from producing potentially lethal amounts of TNF. It felt as if we were on the cusp of a big find, poised to unlock a previously unrecognized mechanism by which the brain prevented inflammation. Figuring out how CNI-1493 in the brain worked to block TNF in the bloodstream held the key to unlocking useful information to make new drugs, and devices, to inhibit inflammation. I was convinced that the brain amplified the effects of very low levels of CNI-1493 and then sent out a signal to the peripheral tissues to turn off TNF synthesis. This extraordinary system seemed to rest on a hair trigger, with the default position set to off, so that the brain could process even a very tiny signal from a molecule like CNI-1493 and broadcast a widespread message that shut down TNF throughout the body. But how?

Under the heavy influence of classic textbook teaching, we looked first in the likeliest place: the bloodstream. The brain controls blood hormones via the pituitary gland, a small, hormone-rich organ on a stalk, dangling from the base of the brain. Situated in a sinus just behind the nose, it receives input from the brain which causes it to release hormones into the blood that control the adrenals and other glands. The scientific and medical literature was full of suggestions that the pituitary gland was the major method for the brain's control of the immune response. The pituitary releases ACTH, a hormone that regulates the release of adrenal steroids; the adrenal steroids in turn suppress the immune system and block TNF release. When we measured the levels of pituitary and adrenal hormones, however, we found that they were not influenced by CNI-1493. Our experiments had thus shown that this was not the answer, because pituitary and adrenal functions were not required for CNI-1493 to be effective. Another explanation was needed.

We rehashed, discussed, debated, and puzzled over this problem at our weekly lab meetings. For months we talked around and around the problem, in the hallways, at the wipe boards, in conference rooms, at the bench, and over lunch. We consumed a lot of turkey sandwiches and pizza trying to make sense of what in retrospect lay right before our eyes. We were burdened by the dogma of previous teachings, and stymied in our ability to generate a theory that both explained the results we had seen and could also be subjected to direct experimental proof. In the midst of one such meeting I was suddenly struck by the possibility that the brain did not need the bloodstream to control the immune system, it could use nerves. Typically, in hindsight it now seems obvious, but the idea took us by complete surprise.

Arising from the center of the brain is an evolutionarily ancient nerve that travels to all the major organs of the immune system, a nerve tasked with regulating organ function under the control of the brain. Named the vagus nerve, from the Latin word for "wander," it takes a meandering course, traveling to all the TNF-producing organs. It is best known as a regulator of organ function in the heart and bowels. Now we wondered whether, just perhaps, the vagus nerve might control the immune system from minute to minute as well. Could it be the high-speed cable from the command-and-control center to the immune system through which orders are issued and relayed with speeds nearly unimaginable when compared with the pace of cytokines floating along in the bloodstream? The difference in transmission speed would be like the difference between an electronic instant message and a carrier pigeon. It was hard to think of a more effective way for the brain to retain control from minute to minute. After all, there are countless examples of the brain operating as a high-speed controller—for instance, in deploying messages through nerves with unimaginable rapidity to direct the fine fingertip movements of the concert violinist. Perhaps it could quickly and efficiently regulate the frontline immune cells using neural signals in the vagus nerve.

Since this was a novel idea, not just for us but for immunology in general, we began by turning to the scientific literature for related studies to support or refute the concept. This search led to a captivating saga that took us back several hundred years. For centuries doctors, monks, shamans, priests, acupuncturists, and laymen believed that an individual's state of mind influenced his health. The idea was ancient. Many had proposed that the immune system, as the gatekeeper and front line of host defense, might be the recipient of this mind or brain influence. Bewilderingly, classical immunology had avoided confronting these questions, for reasons clearly elucidated in 1981 by immunologist Robert A. Good: "Immunologists are often asked whether the state of mind can influence the body's defenses. Can positive attitude, a constructive frame of mind, grief, depression, or anxiety alter ability to resist infections, allergies, autoimmunities, or even cancer? Such questions leave me with a feeling of inadequacy because I know deep down that such influences exist, but I am unable to tell how they work, nor can I in any scientific way prescribe how to harness these influences, predict, or control them. Thus they cannot usually be addressed in scientific perspective. In the face of this inadequacy, most immunologists are naturally uneasy and usually plead not to be bothered with such things."[24]

Despite this caveat, a few scientific pioneers had provided some proof in animals that the state of mind can influence an immune response. As far back as 1926, Metal'nikov and Chorine had performed experiments in animals using Pavlovian conditioning to demonstrate that when an external stimulus (like a bell) was repeatedly paired with administration of an immunologically active material (like bacterial extracts), the animals became conditioned or trained to develop an immune response to the external stimulus alone. This phenomenon has been reproduced by dozens of investigators over a period of nearly 80 years. Despite this history, it was a theory that, like the embarrassing uncle who shows up uninvited at every family barbeque, had not achieved general acceptance in immunology. It was flawed because it could not be fully explained. The story lacked a basic map or wiring diagram to explain how it worked. It is a general tenet of scientific discovery that theories are not accepted, and credit is withheld, until the entire story is explained and the mechanism delineated. We allowed ourselves the luxury of wondering whether our ability to unravel the secrets of CNI-1493 in the brain might assuage Robert Good's concerns, and provide a wiring diagram for this part of the immune system.

Our literature searches also uncovered the classic, groundbreaking work of J. Edwin Blalock, who recognized in the 1970s that the immune system and nervous system used common molecules to communicate.[25] This revolutionary finding revealed that the two systems could communicate bidirectionally, using a common set of molecules and receptors to signal information across systems. Neurons produce molecules to transmit information not only to other neurons but also to macrophages and other inflammatory cells; immune cells secrete cytokines and other molecules that can bind to receptors on neurons, which in turn can respond. Blalock proposed a revolutionary and beautifully simple concept, perceived by many at the time as heretical, that the functions of the immune system were not limited to the classical functions of host defense and inflammation: it might also operate like a sensory organ, capable of detecting bacteria, viruses, antigens, tumor cells, and other miniature invaders.

Blalock called this our sixth sense, even suggesting that it is a necessary companion to our five senses because it is critically important that we are able "to be cognizant not only of things we can see, feel, taste, touch, and smell but also those things we cannot." Blalock proposed that the immune system recognized pathogenic molecules and cells and then, like sensory nerve endings in the eye or nose, immediately notified the brain about the status of these "noncognitive stimuli." This process was efficient and effective because the information was transmitted to the brain via the bidirectional, shared molecular language. This concept elicited still more debate, and the volume of the arguments increased as the discussions turned to individuals who were somehow "aware" that they had developed a serious medical problem or infection, even before noticeable signs or symptoms of the disease had expressed themselves. Could these folks simply be more sensitive to their sixth sense? Maybe those who had allegedly forecast their fate, even their own death, were aware of a lot of bad news from their immune system.

Then there were intriguing reports from Linda Watkins, at the University of Colorado in Boulder, who had become interested in the immune system's role in causing disease. She studied "sickness syndrome," a stereotypical hallmark of infection throughout the animal kingdom. As I mentioned previously, afflicted animals, including humans, develop immobility, lethargy, food avoidance, fever, anorexia, sexual inactivity, and depression. Watkins, a psychologist by training, realized that the brain controlled the development of all of these signs and symptoms, but she wondered whether the brain was the primary source of the syndrome, or whether it was responding to signals from the immune system. She reasoned that the brain might well use its extensive sensory neural network to detect the presence of foreign products or cytokines throughout the body, and she devised an ingenious set of experiments.

Professor Watkins administered low levels of either bacterial endotoxin or a cytokine (IL-1) into the abdomen of rats, then cut their vagus nerve, a major conduit that transmits messages along sensory nerves from the visceral organs to the brain. The results were striking: cutting the vagus nerve prevented the development of fever and sickness syndrome. The explanation was at once simple and clear: the vagus nerve transmitted information about the degree of inflammation within the immune system directly to the brain. This was powerful evidence that the brain could respond via the sixth sense to incoming neural input about the status of inflammation in the abdomen, and presumably other peripheral tissues. When this flow of neural information was disrupted—in this case by cutting the vagus nerve—the rat's brain did not "know" that it should direct the onset of the sickness syndrome. The question was answered: the immune system, by releasing cytokines, normally instructs the brain to cause the signs and symptoms of disease. This was further validation of the cytokine theory of disease, but with a twist: it moved the brain, and its projection, the vagus nerve, onto center stage.

Watkins's work, like many other revolutionary discoveries, was not widely acknowledged or appreciated until much later. In part her results were not completely understood, because classic teaching about the vagus nerve had focused on its roles in regulating the function of the standard visceral organs, like the heart, rather than the immune system. The vagus nerve originates in the brain stem, travels down through the neck, and splits into branch after branch, eventually touching every vital organ. It is a major conduit from the brain that modulates heart rate variability, respiratory rate, and thousands of other unseen functions. The vagus nerve is a hardwired component of subconscious brain function that is like a neural superhighway enabling the brain to regulate the finest details of specific organ function.

One of the best studied vagus nerve pathways involves the regulation of heart rate. Your heart normally beats 72 times a minute or so, but these beats do not occur at a fixed, constant rate. There is a variability to the healthy heart rate; each beat occurs a little faster or a little slower than the one before; the time between individual heartbeats varies, a measurable response that is termed instantaneous heart rate variability. Over time, your average number of heartbeats per minute may be 72, but the interval between heartbeats constantly changes. This "flexible component" of human heart rate is a sign of health; the more flexibility the better. Heart rate variability is controlled by the vagus nerve: high levels of instantaneous heart rate variability are a sign of high vagus nerve activity.

The vagus nerve proper is composed of thousands of thin nerve fibers that travel to the target organs. Neurons within these fibers terminate in the organs, where they release the molecule acetylcholine. Acetylcholine is a neurotransmitter, so called because it functions as a specific chemical signaling agent. Acetylcholine is released only when the brain transmits a specific electrical signal to the nerve ending, telling it to release the molecule. The nerve ending does not release acetylcholine into the bloodstream but into a narrow space between the nerve ending itself and the adjacent cell. The released acetylcholine binds to a specific docking station, or receptor, on specific recipient cells. In the heart, for example, acetylcholine released by the vagus nerve binds to specific receptors on cells whose job it is to increase the time interval between adjacent heartbeats. Thus, when the vagus nerve fires, it releases acetylcholine near these cells, which sop it up and respond by instantaneously slowing the heart rate. When the vagus nerve is quiet, acetylcholine is not released, and the heart rate transiently speeds up. This cycling activity of the vagus nerve in releasing acetylcholine causes variability in instantaneous heart rate; the changes in beat-to-beat interval are dependent on the vagus nerve's activity.

The release of acetylcholine in the region of the heart's pacemaker cells establishes the time until the next heartbeat. Healthy, you remain blissfully unaware of all this activity; it is beneath the radar of your consciousness, working all the time, regulating the function of your heart. You may not have fully appreciated your own vagus nerve, lying right there in your neck next to your carotid artery, but don't underestimate it. It is on permanent call, 24-7-365, ready to modulate your cardiac efficiency and heartbeat. With this background on the activity of the vagus nerve, we can go on to discuss the finding that parasympathetic signals, in the form of acetylcholine released by vagus nerve endings, precisely suppress the immune system's production of cytokines.

At the time that we began to study the role of the vagus nerve in controlling cytokine release, it was a foreign concept that the brain, itself a mass of nerves and neural pathways, would use nerves to control the immune response. Centuries of scientific study had focused primarily on interactions between molecules floating in the bloodstream as the major controllers of the immune response to infection. It was stunning to even consider that a neural pathway could explain how the body is protected from excessive TNF release. Scientific reductionism of complex physiological events had provided a clear understanding of how the brain's connections to specific organs through the vagus nerve could control functions, such as heart rate, insulin output, and gastrointestinal motility. With rare exceptions, however, the vagus nerve connection to the immune system was not included in this classical list.

This entrenched belief had its origins in the humoral theory of immunity. Blood-borne molecules, or so it was thought, provided all the necessary messages about the nature of the threat, the magnitude of the immune response, and the stage of the inflammatory process; all you needed to control and regulate the immune system were the circulating or humoral factors, not nerves. But in biological terms this humoral, or blood-borne, system operated at a snail's pace, restricted by the time it took for the molecules to travel from their site of origin to the location of the responding cells at the local site of infection. Bacterial toxins, cytokines, and steroids each interact with macrophages, T cells, B cells, and the other cellular components of the immune system. Sailing leisurely through the bloodstream, molecules produced by bacteria or the immune cells eventually meet an appropriate receptor on a responding cell, which triggers or modulates inflammation.

Thinking it through, we realized that humoral signaling was nothing at all like the nearly instantaneous, hair-trigger regulation that can be provided by neural signals. There had to be a faster way for the brain's command-and-control center to supervise the activity on the front lines. Why should it rely on schooners to carry messages to the front when it had ready access to high-speed Internet connections, installed and ready to go? Moreover, a neural mechanism in control of the immune system would provide a method for the brain to selectively signal the immune cells in the liver, for example, without sending the same signal to the right hand. This selectivity is not possible with humoral factors, because elevated levels of steroids in the bloodstream will of necessity cause comparable effects on cells residing in both locations. It would be like sending the same battle orders to all fronts in a war. It makes sense that the command-and-control center should be able to send specific signals to specific regions of the battle; this could be readily accomplished using messages in nerves rather than the bloodstream.

The immune system is widely distributed throughout the body's organs. The vast majority of the macrophages, mast cells, and dendritic cells that make potentially lethal amounts of TNF and HMGB1 are disseminated throughout the spleen, liver, lungs, kidneys, bone marrow, intestines, thymus, and lymph nodes. All of these sites receive input from the vagus nerve. If one were to engineer a system to prevent these macrophages from releasing lethal amounts of cytokines, the vagus nerve would seem to be an ideal place to start. It is a vitally important nerve that could instantaneously shut down the immune response, prevent the release of TNF and HMGB1, and prevent the development of septic shock or severe sepsis. By using the network of nerves in the vagus nerve system, the brain could easily command one response in the liver, and an entirely different one in the spleen.

MANHASSET, LONG ISLAND, MAY 1998. Every scientist thinks up lots of experiments—an unreasonable number actually, more than he could accomplish in even several lifetimes. On a typical day in a busy lab, at least three or four new ideas are hatched before lunch, proliferating like rabbits overrunning the available resources. Not all the ideas can be tested. Prioritization is a necessity, and some experimental ideas are inevitably moved to the back burner, where they simmer out of the way of the daily stress of managing a research team and writing grants to pay the lab's bills. But I remember clearly the day we conceived of the experiment to test directly whether the vagus nerve controlled the immune system.

A group of us were sitting around the conference table in the windowless boardroom on the fourth floor of the Boas Marks Research Building. The tabletop was littered with picked-over pizza boxes, and half the team struggled in the effort to fight off their postprandial urge to sleep. We had just reviewed some results of injecting CNI-1493 into the brain of rats, and I said, "If CNI-1493 works by activating the vagus nerve to fire, and the release of acetylcholine in the immune system turns off TNF, then we should be able to turn off TNF by applying an electrical signal to the vagus nerve." The thought was at once exciting and simple. I jumped up to the wipe board and quickly sketched a diagram connecting the brain to the immune system via the vagus nerve. It suddenly seemed so obvious that we thought it must be true. That night, I woke up at 3 a.m. convinced that this idea could not only explain the increased susceptibility some patients have to inflammatory disease, but guide the development of therapies to switch off excessive cytokine release. It was also clear that this neural control of cytokine production would not be limited to TNF but include other cytokines as well. Much later, this proved to be the case, because the vagus nerve pathway can indeed also switch off HMGB1 production.

The next day I went to the operating room of my hospital, talked one of the anesthesiologists out of a used handheld battery-operated nerve stimulator, and brought it back to the lab. When we applied the electrical stimulator to the vagus nerve in rats, the results were clear: vagus nerve stimulation significantly blocked the release of TNF. The vagus nerve could control the immune response and prevent lethal amounts of TNF from being produced. Here was a previously unknown mechanism by which the brain could reflexively monitor and adjust the inflammatory response during infection or injury. I called this neural loop the inflammatory reflex because it functions like a knee-jerk reflex. In the knee jerk, or "patellar reflex," the doctor's rubber hammer stretches the patellar tendon to elicit a rapidly opposing motor action in the quadriceps muscle. In the inflammatory reflex, the vagus nerve is "stretched," or stimulated, by inflammatory molecules and then fires an opposing "anti-inflammatory" signal to prevent further inflammation.

The inflammatory reflex is both fast and subconscious, an elegantly protective mechanism to prevent injury caused by an excessive immune response. Our new theory predicted that if outflow through the vagus nerve was diminished, as is known to occur during critical illness and chronic inflammatory disease, it might actually facilitate the immune system, fostering excessive TNF release. The immune system is normally poised to unleash a fatal sequence of cytokines, like an attack dog straining furiously at the chain that holds it back from the pedestrians gazing through the fence. The vagus nerve was the chain on the dog. What happened if it snapped? I found myself thinking back to Janice, wondering if this explained why she had suddenly developed first septic shock and then severe sepsis. Had her nervous system failed her when she needed it most?

The vagus nerve, like other nerves, carries information from the brain in the form of a specialized electrical current made up of action potentials, which are propagated along the length of the nerve until they arrive at the nerve endings. Vagus nerve endings are packed with tiny vesicles, each chock-full of acetylcholine. The acetylcholine molecules are released every time an action potential arrives at the nerve ending. The acetylcholine is released into a narrow space between the nerve ending and the cells that are under the nerve's control. This narrow space, called a synapse, is like a small creek running between the nerve and the cells it controls. The electrical signal in the nerve cannot jump across the creek to the other side, so instead the nerve sends acetylcholine to cross the creek, like putting a message into a canoe and shoving it across to a recipient awaiting information. Once the acetylcholine reaches the other bank of the creek, it inserts itself into specific docks located on the responding cells. Our experiments showed that it was possible for acetylcholine to insert itself onto macrophages and regulate the immune system. In this case, the signal in the canoe (acetylcholine) docked on responding cells on the other bank (receptors on macrophages) that in turn switched off the release of TNF.

I termed this ability of the vagus nerve to control cytokine release the "cholinergic anti-inflammatory pathway," to highlight the potential importance of acetylcholine-like molecules as normal constituents of the protective anti-inflammatory response to infection or injury. This concept predicted that if the vagus nerve, or perhaps the brain's control over the vagus nerve, ever became dysfunctional, then TNF release would be unfettered, a situation that would cause shock and tissue injury. This function of the vagus nerve as a "master off switch" on the immune system would normally suppress an excessive inflammatory response. If for some reason it failed to suppress the response, the results could be catastrophic. We immediately began to consider how to make molecules that we could administer as drugs. By producing molecules that would bind to the acetylcholine receptor or dock on macrophages, it should be possible to block TNF release at will.

MAY 2000. We published a paper in *Nature* describing our discovery that vagus nerve stimulation can suppress TNF release and prevent lethal shock and tissue injury. By stimulating the vagus nerve with an electrode, we could effectively prevent the immune system from producing shock-inducing and organ-damaging amounts of TNF in the blood. Stimulation of the vagus nerve also prevented excessive TNF synthesis in experimental conditions in animals with lesser degrees of inflammation, including arthritis caused by administering an irritant into the hind paw. The converse scenario also proved true: we found that cutting the vagus nerve (vagotomy) *increased* the TNF response to endotoxin. Rats subjected to vagotomy made significantly more TNF because we had disrupted the braking mechanism of the nerve on cytokine production. In rodents at least, it was clear that an intact vagus nerve and normally functioning cholinergic nervous system were required to prevent the highly dangerous release of TNF during bacterial infection.

I recalled those days in May 1985 when Janice survived her episode of septic shock. She had survived in part because of medical devices including respirators, dialysis machines, intravenous pumps, and cardiac monitors. Since then the medical armamentarium has added dozens more devices that support the lives of the critically ill, including an artificial heart and deep-brain stimulators. Amazingly, vagus nerve stimulators have also been developed as a treatment for epilepsy, and they have proved to be quite safe. Might they be useful in patients like Janice as a method to prevent a sudden, potentially lethal TNF surge? Or perhaps it would be possible to develop a drug that takes the place of acetylcholine, a chemical that we could administer into the veins, where it could find the macrophage receptor for acetylcholine and switch off TNF synthesis.

JANUARY 2001. We set out next to identify the specific receptor molecule on the macrophage that turned off the TNF, hoping that if we discovered its molecular fingerprint, we would be able to design and develop medicinal molecules that blocked inflammation. There are dozens of closely related acetylcholine receptors on neurons and other cells, but the acetylcholine receptor type on macrophages was unknown. This made the task of isolating the specific receptor subtype on macrophages a complicated endeavor. After months of searching through the possible acetylcholine candidate genes and proteins in macrophages, we eventually found that the pattern of receptor expression was most consistent with a molecule known as alpha-7.[26] The final proof that alpha-7 was the critical macrophage acetylcholine receptor came from our studies of mice that lacked all their alpha-7 genes. These mice had been genetically engineered to delete the alpha-7 gene, a technique referred to by molecular biologists as the alpha-7 knockout.

Macrophages from these knock-out mice, which lacked alpha-7, continued to produce TNF at normal rates, even in the presence of acetylcholine, indicating that alpha-7 was required for acetylcholine to inhibit TNF. More striking still, when we electrically stimulated the vagus nerve of the alpha-7 knock-out mice, they continued to produce high levels of TNF. The inescapable conclusion was that the product of a single gene encoding alpha-7 was absolutely required for the vagus nerve to suppress the acute immune response. This analysis had confirmed that the entire cholinergic anti-inflammatory system converged on a single gene product expressed by macrophages, and perhaps other immune cells, to turn off TNF. The inflammatory reflex was dependent on neural signals transmitted to immune cells via the vagus nerve in order to achieve effective protection against cytokine toxicity. It was as if macrophages on the front lines all had the same decoder. It processed incoming messages from the command-and-control center, causing them all to turn off cytokine release.

JANUARY 2003. We published the identity of alpha-7 as an anti-inflammatory macrophage receptor in *Nature*, in a paper that attracted a great deal of attention to the possibility of producing drugs that would act through this pathway. It was a thrilling time because we could clearly envision therapeutic possibilities for controlling the pathological action of TNF. It seemed quite likely that we could develop alternative therapies with molecules that would target the alpha-7 receptor to turn off TNF synthesis. My colleague Luis Ulloa recently completed the final scientific piece of the story, connecting the cholinergic anti-inflammatory pathway to TNF and HMGB1 by proving that acetylcholine can suppress the release of HMGB1 by macrophages. Thinking back to Janice's case, it all made sense. It is quite possible that decreased activity in her vagus nerve failed to suppress her immune system, which therefore responded excessively to a relatively small number of unseen bacteria. During her first episode of immune activation, her impaired brain may have failed to send the needed blocking signals to her immune system to prevent the sudden release of TNF, so she developed acute septic shock. During her second episode of immune activation, the cholinergic anti-inflammatory pathway may have failed to prevent the release of HMGB1, and she therefore developed severe sepsis.

Twenty years later, I cannot know for sure, but the evidence available today indicates that this is a plausible explanation for why some patients with bacterial infection develop acute septic shock, some develop severe sepsis, and others develop neither. The failure of this command-and-control system may occur inside the brain, and we have already seen that brain dysfunction is an integral part of critical illness. But the system can also break down at a number of other locations. For example, the macrophages may become altered during the immune response, either as a direct effect of being activated or because they have been exposed to other cytokines and hormones, which may reduce the macrophages' ability to respond to alpha-7 so that they fail to heed the signals from the vagus nerve. Neural signals within the voluntary nervous system control every movement of your fingers and toes, and signals within the involuntary nervous system control every beat of your heart. The theory of the cholinergic anti-inflammatory pathway indicates that the vagus nerve, by controlling the magnitude of the immune system's response to germs, is also critical in protecting us from developing acute septic shock, severe sepsis, and other diseases caused by excessive cytokine production.

Thousands of patients in hospitals and intensive care units become infected with bacteria every day. Countless hospital admissions are the result of infections that develop at home as pneumonia, appendicitis, diverticulitis, or other problems. Millions of cases of infection run an uncomplicated course that does not lead to either acute septic shock or severe sepsis. The immune system responds appropriately to the infection, and, with antibiotics and other medicines, the germs are eradicated and the patient recovers. The cytokine response activated by the bacteria is effectively switched off by the vagus nerve. The cytokine response can cause fever, aching muscles, and a sickness syndrome with anorexia and fatigue, and as the cytokine levels return to normal, the patients go on to recover uneventfully, returning to health, home, and normalcy. The inflammatory reflex protects most of these patients from their own immune response by limiting the amount of cytokines produced. But some are not so lucky, and for them a few bacteria cause things to go terribly wrong. If the vagus nerve falls asleep at the switch, the same bacteria can trigger an overwhelming TNF or HMGB1 response leading to acute septic shock, organ damage, severe sepsis, and perhaps death.

If you were to visit the intensive care unit of a major medical center, you would see as you walked through the long line of beds that nearly every patient has a Foley catheter draining the urinary bladder into a plastic bag at the bedside. Most patients will be on a respirator, many will have surgical wounds, and nearly all will have intravenous and-or intra-arterial catheters, all portals for bacterial invasion. Acute septic shock, or even severe sepsis, does not occur in all of these patients. Although at present we do not fully understand what causes some of them to suddenly unleash their TNF or HMGB1, it is clear that the vagus nerve can be a crucial controller of this response.

The majority of people who develop acute septic shock or

severe sepsis have overt brain dysfunction, the most common manifestations of which are confusion, delirium, and weakness. Mortality from severe sepsis is twice as high in patients whose mental status is abnormal as in patients with no evidence of brain dysfunction. Critically ill patients with severe sepsis usually develop multiple signs of brain dysfunction, including autonomic dysregulation,[27] hypothalamic-pituitary dysfunction, and accelerated metabolic rates. It is as if the thermostatic functions of the command center become overloaded or short-circuited. Regulation of body temperature is impaired, and the patients develop fever or hypothermia. The normal vagus nerve–controlled regulation of heart rate is altered. Instead of a variable or flexible interval between heartbeats, their heartbeats march along in lockstep, invariable, a condition associated with significantly higher mortality rates than those of patients with normal heart rate variability.

I believe that abnormal or diminished activity in the vagus nerve control of the immune system can lead to uncontrolled, excessive cytokine release. Diminution in the activity of the cholinergic anti-inflammatory pathway would favor the overproduction of TNF, HMGB1, and other inflammatory mediators, perhaps to levels that can become toxic and dangerous to survival. Depressed brain function may be a proximal cause of the overproduction of cytokines that injures the patient.

Failure within the cholinergic anti-inflammatory pathway can occur at a number of points along it. It is possible that the higher brain structures that control vagus nerve outflow might become unresponsive to the sensory input normally provided by the immune system. For example, if the sensory nerves, which normally detect the presence of cytokines in the tissues, fail to signal the brain properly, then the inflammatory reflex will not be activated. In that case, absent a descending "off" signal in the vagus nerve, cytokine release would proceed, unimpeded, until toxicity developed. This might be likened to a state of immune "sensory deprivation," because the central nervous system is not aware of the inflammation in the body.

Another possibility is that depressed output in the vagus nerve, and a resultant increase in cytokine synthesis, is sufficient to cause a damaging inflammatory response to an otherwise innocuous infection or injury. An example of this may be found in patients with arthritis or other autoimmune diseases who have abnormally low activity in their vagus nerve. In these cases it is plausible that diminished vagus nerve signals enable excessive cytokine release, which in turn drives inflammatory damage in the joints.

Finally, it is theoretically possible for the system to fail even when the vagus nerve is intact. For example, if the cells of the immune system become resistant to the effects of acetylcholine, then macrophages may continue to produce high levels of TNF or HMGB1 even in the presence of an active vagus nerve. There is precedent for this scenario in the nervous system, because repetitive stimulation of a neural pathway causes the response to diminish with time, a process known as desensitization, or tachyphylaxis. Tachyphylaxis within the cholinergic anti-inflammatory pathway would predictably lead to an overproduction of cytokines, causing organ injury or damage.

Today's "classic teaching," which is undoubtedly true, is that severe sepsis and septic shock can impair brain function. But I also believe that sometimes brain impairment or impairment of the cholinergic anti-inflammatory pathway can occur first, which in turn facilitates or causes the overproduction of cytokines. Dysfunction within the cholinergic anti-inflammatory pathway could be an underlying or contributing cause of the excessive cytokine production that causes severe sepsis or septic shock. The broadest implications of the cholinergic anti-inflammatory pathway lead one to consider whether it might fulfill, as J. Edwin Blalock said, "the final challenge in Dr. Good's narrative by finding a way to harness an influence of the brain over the immune system . . . Bringing these ideas to fruition may now provide a means for harnessing the possibly powerful influences of the CNS over the immune system."[28] This new knowledge of the cholinergic anti-inflammatory pathway has already provided some surprising insights into both physiological pathways and therapeutic strategies to prevent excessive cytokine release and inflammation. It is significant that some of these strategies lend themselves directly to human testing, either to prevent the acute overproduction of shock-inducing amounts of cytokines during critical illness, or to control cytokine during chronic diseases such as arthritis, inflammatory bowel disease, and other diseases of excessive cytokine activity.

ten

Legacy

I have tried to tell Janice's story to illustrate the science of shock and sepsis, but it is my story too. Most doctors don't attend the funerals of their patients. Some do, I know, and more probably should, but I did not attend Janice's funeral. I should have gone as a kind gesture to a devastated family. Guilt, denial, an overwhelming sense of a failure, and an inability to understand what had really happened all kept me away. Maybe I could have explained to someone there that I really did not know why Janice died and neither did my colleagues. All the sophisticated language, medical explanations, and intensive therapies that were thrown into the septic mix, into the faces of the suffering family, and into the veins and heart of the little girl, were inadequate. I should have attended for selfish reasons, because perhaps the nightmares would have stopped sooner, those nightly visions of Janice's failed code. I should have gone to see Janice's little coffin.

Since Janice's death we have made significant progress in our ability to treat acute septic shock and severe sepsis. Although there is no single "magic bullet" to cure them, there have been discrete, incremental advances that have somewhat improved the odds of surviving. These include new guidelines for delivering intravenous fluids that can improve survival for patients admitted to the emergency room with acute septic shock. There are newer, more powerful imaging techniques including magnetic resonance imaging (MRI) and computed tomography (CT) scanning technology that can reveal in minute detail the presence of previously unseen infections hidden deep in the major organs, diagnostic tools that were simply unimaginable in Janice's time. There is a new drug, "activated protein C," which has been approved by the FDA for use in patients with severe sepsis. It can benefit some severe sepsis patients, in some perhaps by slowing coagulation at sites of inflammation or organ damage, and in others perhaps by suppressing the production of some cytokines. There are new guidelines for the use of respirators, based on the discovery that the ventilation pressure can stimulate the lungs to release cytokines that may cause damage in other organs. There is renewed attention to monitoring blood sugar, and administering insulin in order to keep glucose levels under tight control. As of this writing, there are studies in progress to determine whether a combination of these improved therapeutic approaches will together reduce the mortality of severe sepsis. There is also universal agreement that much more is still needed, and that the ideal treatments would be based on a better understanding of the causes of severe sepsis.

There are no highly visible patient action groups, no coalitions of septic shock or severe sepsis survivors, no political action committees, and no unified objective among people addressing severe sepsis today. It is striking that fewer dollars have been spent on research for sepsis than for less prevalent diseases whose advocates have a unified front and are politically organized. I believe that in the future we will reduce the death rate of acute septic shock and severe sepsis. This drives me and my colleagues to study how cytokines such as TNF and HMGB1 cause disease, and how the brain regulates their effects. I envision that one day we will have drugs that act like acetylcholine to safely restrain the immune response. There may well be computer-driven pacemakers that function in the place of the brain and the vagus nerve when they are disabled, to keep us safe from ourselves. I believe that in the future the intensivists will be able to select from a panel of drugs based on the principles of the cytokine theory of disease.

One possible approach is to activate neural anti-inflammatory mechanisms using small molecules that initiate signals in the brain, upstream of the vagus nerve. As I write, the search is on to identify drugs that specifically switch off inflammation. If this hunt is successful, I envision a family of "psychoactive vagus nerve stimulators," pills that suppress inflammation in the peripheral organs by causing the brain to turn on the vagus nerve. Support for this approach has come from surprising places because there is solid evidence that several widely used anti-inflammatory drugs can also function as "pharmacological vagus nerve stimulators." This list includes the nonsteroidal anti-inflammatory drugs aspirin, indomethacin, and ibuprofen, each of which has been reported to substantially increase vagus nerve activity. I now suspect that some of the clinical benefit from these drugs may be due to their activity in stimulating the cholinergic anti-inflammatory pathway in the vagus nerve.

Another therapeutic approach for the future may be to directly stimulate the vagus nerve with an electrical device, similar to what we have already done in animal experiments. This is not as far-fetched as it may seem at first blush, because more than 10,000 patients with epilepsy have already been treated with an implanted vagus nerve stimulator, like a pacemaker for the vagus nerve, as treatment for their seizures. Vagus nerve stimulation with these small devices (implanted in the upper chest) is remarkably safe and well tolerated. The immunological effects of this approach are being studied now, and we await the results with interest to assess whether stimulating the vagus nerve in humans modulates cytokine synthesis and the development of inflammation.

I imagine a bedside device, at the ready in the intensive care unit, which can be applied to the patient as needed to manipulate the cytokine response. The output settings of this theoretical device would be guided by the individual patient's cytokine response measured in real time. These levels would be projected onto a screen showing the cytokine pattern in the tissues, like an EKG monitor for the immune system. This complex cytokine data would be stored and processed in computers that track the results to identify patterns that can be manipulated and controlled. This approach might be aided by tracking software not unlike what the military uses to pick out an incoming missile from a massive collection of confusing radar images.

Besides implantable devices, it should also be possible to develop pharmacological agents that target the peripheral alpha-7 macrophage receptor to inhibit synthesis and release of TNF and HMGB1. There is already an important precedent for this approach in humans with ulcerative colitis, an inflammatory bowel disease that can in some cases be treated effectively with nicotine. It is not yet known whether the clinical benefit of nicotine occurred because nicotine acted via alpha-7 to inhibit cytokine synthesis, but that is a reasonable and now testable hypothesis. We and others have completed preclinical studies using cholinergic agents to block excessive inflammation in standard animal models of diabetes, arthritis, septic shock, and sepsis.

It may also be possible to achieve some control over excessive cytokine production without the use of either drugs or devices but through conscious modulation of the patient's own immune response. It is theoretically possible now through biofeedback to "teach" people to increase their own cholinergic anti-inflammatory pathway to suppress their cytokine production. For obvious reasons, it is highly unlikely that this approach will be applicable to severely injured patients with impaired ability to think. But I can readily envision applying these principles to chronic illnesses characterized by excessive cytokine release in clearheaded, mentally functional patients, such as those with rheumatoid arthritis and inflammatory bowel disease.

In these diseases there is clear evidence that excessive cytokine production is the cause. The cytokine levels are not high enough to cause shock, and the patients do not have brain dysfunction, so it may well be possible one day to use biofeedback to increase vagus nerve activity and decrease cytokine production in the inflamed tissues. Biofeedback can be used to train patients to slow their own heart rate, an effect that functionally increases the activity in the vagus nerve. It is not yet known whether the increased vagus nerve firing to the heart will also suppress the release of TNF and HMGB1 by the immune system, but it is a possibility that is being studied now.

Interestingly, trained athletes have extremely high vagus nerve activity with slow heart rates and high beat-to-beat variability. These same individuals may be protected against chronic inflammatory diseases, perhaps because they live in a state of high vagus output that would predictably suppress the toxicity of their immune system. A powerful stimulus for increasing vagus nerve output is controlled breathing exercises combined with aerobic exercise training. There is solid evidence that some professional athletes are at peak efficiency when they function in *between their heartbeats*. Successful biathlon sharpshooters fire between heartbeats, and some professional baseball players and golfers actually strike the ball between heart-beats, when their hearts are still. This is accomplished by increasing vagus nerve output at the time of peak performance, which instantaneously slows the heart at the critical moment of function or impact. It's possible that "being in the zone" is a state of high vagus output. Increased output can also provide maximal protection against the toxicity of an inflammatory response that occurs with vigorous exercise, muscle tears, and ligament strains.

Hypnosis, meditation, and prayer can each significantly increase vagus nerve output and inhibit immediate-type and delayed-type hypersensitivity responses in humans. Similarly, exercise, biofeedback training, and acupuncture have each been used to modulate vagus nerve activity and to reduce experimental inflammation. "Positive affect" and "states of mind" have been linked to higher levels of protective antibody responses to vaccination, and to protection against viruses that cause the common cold. Historically, the earliest studies that addressed the relationship between the nervous system and the inflammatory response were based on training and conditioning to alter an intra-abdominal inflammatory process. Behavioral conditioning and learned association have been shown to influence acute inflammatory responses and alter the course of inflammation in humans.

These approaches have not been widely embraced, however, in part because it has not been clear how they work. Scientific uncertainty about the mechanistic basis for these effects has hampered attempts to optimize and standardize the approaches. It is now possible to consider whether these approaches influence the cholinergic anti-inflammatory pathway, and whether this can provide a new avenue to explore these methods. One can envision studies in volunteers in which behavioral conditioning and learned associations are paired with vagus nerve activity to improve the ability to monitor training sessions and effectiveness by measuring heart rate variability and cytokine responses.

Another approach is to consider whether patients with depressed vagus nerve activity are at increased risk for inflammatory disease. Indeed, there is abundant, solid clinical evidence that autonomic dysfunction and depressed vagus nerve activity go hand in hand with the development of chronic human inflammatory diseases in association with cytokine overproduction. Autonomic dysfunction occurs in rheumatoid arthritis, diabetes, and other autoimmune disorders. It was believed to be a secondary result or complication of the inflammatory disease, but the new insights provided by the cholinergic anti-inflammatory pathway make it plausible to consider the alternative possibility: that decreased vagus nerve activity may actually be a contributing cause of the development of inflammation. In other words, a depression of vagus nerve activity is like a brake failure that unleashes excessive or uncontrolled cytokine responses. Autonomic dysfunction can be detected via abnormal blood pressure responses when a subject lying flat is suddenly tilted upright. It may also be a sign that the cholinergic anti-inflammatory pathway is impaired, leading to cytokine overproduction that is a disease hallmark. If this is indeed the case, then increasing vagus nerve activity using either a training paradigm or drug may provide a therapeutic advantage.

We have seen that critical illness in humans is inevitably associated with severe brain dysfunction, and it is appropriate to consider whether this is caused by the disease as a result of diminished brain perfusion and the accumulation of circulating toxins that depress neuronal activity in brain centers controlling consciousness. But the alternate theory also may well be true, that critical illness in humans develops because of the brain's failure to restrain the immune system. Robert Munford, an infectious-disease physician and the Bromberg Professor of Internal Medicine at the University of Texas Southwestern Medical School in Dallas, has proposed that systemic anti-inflammatory pathways are activated at the earliest stages of an injury or infection, and that the brain plays a powerful role in creating an anti-inflammatory state in the bloodstream. The purpose of this state is to confine the body's inflammatory reaction to the local site where the infection or injury has occurred. The brain drives a major, systemic anti-inflammatory response by activating the adrenals to release glucocorticoids (steroid hormones) and epinephrine (an anti-inflammatory hormone), and the vagus nerve to release acetylcholine. The systemic anti-inflammatory response is the predominant response, so that the pro-inflammatory effects of TNF and HMGB1 at the site of an infection become like a magnet, attracting inflammatory cells to the center of the problem like iron filings.

This theory explains not only the brain's ability to prevent the development of systemic toxicity from excessive TNF and HMGB1 but the fact that critically ill patients who survive for an extended period in this state may develop secondary infections with germs and fungi that normally occur only in patients who have been "immunosuppressed" because of chemotherapy, transplant drugs, or AIDS. Perhaps too much of this brain-derived anti-inflammatory response suppresses the immune system too much. At some point, the brain decreases its anti-inflammatory output, possibly to restore some increased systemic pro-inflammatory activity. It tries to maintain the fragile balance between too much inflammation (that can cause tremendous harm) and not enough (allowing infection). Perhaps in addition to preventing the formation of horrible, painful memories during the illness, depressed brain activity may aid the recovery process. As the brain begins to function again, it will restore the immune system's activity by reducing anti-inflammatory output through the pituitary gland, sympathetic nervous system, and vagus nerve.

We have learned a great deal about what caused Janice to develop septic shock and then severe sepsis, but after more than 20 years, her sudden death is still unexplained. A leading possibility is that severe sepsis damaged her heart. Recent studies of sepsis survivors indicate that even after surviving sepsis and being discharged from the hospital to go home, these patients are at significantly increased risk of dying. The higher death rate among these sepsis survivors may persist for up to five years after discharge; sepsis survivors die at rates up to eight times faster than patients who never developed severe sepsis. By outward appearances, these sepsis survivors had recovered and seemed well. The data suggest otherwise, however, raising the possibility that severe sepsis can cause deep-seated, or at least unresolved or persisting, damage.

Cytokine levels and cholinergic anti-inflammatory pathway activity have not yet been measured in sepsis survivors, but we have recently begun to consider whether abnormalities in these pathways can underlie the increased mortality. We have begun to measure serum HMGB1 levels in survivors of severe sepsis, and surprisingly, even on the day the patients were sent home, their HMGB1 levels remained extremely high, in some cases as high as when the severe sepsis had been at its worst. We do not know whether chronically elevated HMGB1 levels shorten life span, but we are now looking for the answer to this question. We are examining other questions, too: Why is it that TNF and HMGB1 can both cause a chronic inflammatory disease like arthritis? Why do extremely high levels of TNF cause shock? What happens to patients who are exposed to high levels of HMGB1, as in arthritis—do they become immune to its toxicity, and are they protected from developing severe sepsis?

Many of the advances since Janice's time have still not been validated in human clinical trials. Indeed, the major ideas presented here—that TNF is a mediator of acute septic shock, that the vagus nerve can control the immune response, and that HMGB1 may be a mediator of severe sepsis—are still under varying stages of study necessary before attempts can be made to treat human subjects. Years of additional work, costing millions of dollars, are needed before we will know whether treatment based on these ideas can be used to reduce human suffering. It is fair to ask, "What if these trials fail simply because, as far as we have come, we still do not really know enough about TNF, HMGB1, the vagus nerve, and severe sepsis? Have Janice's life and all this work been for nothing?" I believe the answer is no.

Scientific progress that leads to cures comes from stepwise advances, as new ideas are presented, tested, challenged, and revised. Therapies may come from a modification or revision of a theory that has fallen out of favor. Consider that there is still debate about how some of our standard medicines, like aspirin, really work; our knowledge of how it works continues to grow as people take it for their headaches, arthritis, and heart attack. An analogy can be made to antibodies against cytokines. The idea that excessive cytokine release causes disease is now perceived as a relatively simple one, and I cannot predict how the new theories presented here will be viewed in the future. Of course, I hope that clinical trials with anti-HMGB1, and therapeutics based on the vagus nerve, are effective in humans as originally conceived, but only time, and a great deal more work, will answer our questions.

Janice lived 11 short months at home, and one long month in the burn unit. Those who cared for her were touched by her innocence, her gentleness, and the unfairness of it all. Her time at home was probably memorialized in family photos, and the stories exchanged on special days, such as her birthday and the anniversary of her death. Her hospitalization created a legacy of a different sort, one that is very much alive 20 years later. I know that her immune system's fatal sequence burned itself out in four weeks, but I do not like to think of it that way. I find it more reassuring to think that Janice, like an angel, lives on in the efforts to define and understand the nature of the individual cytokines involved in her septic shock and severe sepsis and the way in which her body fought to prevent their release. Her indirect legacy can be found right now in the scientific literature, online at PubMed under the keyword *cytokine*. I like to think of this work as an unfinished mural stretching for miles around a city or large university, being painted around the clock, every day, by students, scientists, and investigators who do not know each other and cannot see each other because the wall is too long. They may not even know what is being painted on the far side, but they are driven to paint perfectly, and finish the job, motivated by their own angels. I am confident that some day, I hope soon, the work will be done, and this mural will be a guidepost for the weary patients and their families awaiting cures for cytokine-based diseases.

Acknowledgments

I am indebted to all those who helped me with this book, generously taking time to read drafts, make suggestions, and talk to me about their experiences with severe sepsis. They are Nancy Ferullo, Vivian Carpenter, Dee Prieto, Jared Huston, Margot Gallowitsch, Richard Goldstein, Andy Feigen, Carl Nathan, Scott Somers, Brett Giroir, Bob Munford, Jan Andersson, Hans-Guistaf Ljunggren, Ursula Weiss, Sharon Tracey Barret, David Sheehan, Father Tom Hartman, Bill Bruce, David Herndon, John Kane, Amy Wilfert, and Jamie Talan. I am very grateful to all my scientific collaborators and research colleagues over the years, and especially to Tony Cerami, Chris Czura, Haichao Wang, Huan Yang, Luis Ulloa, Hong Wang, and Steve Lowry. I am extremely indebted to Shaw Warren, Mitch Fink, John Mountain, and Ulf Andersson for their insights, encouragement, and friendship. To my editor, Dan Gordon, a gifted and thoughtful colleague, whose unique combination of patience and enthusiasm helped enormously. To Jane Nevins, who saw the potential of the book for Dana Press. And finally, to Tricia Tracey, whose love and support is woven into this story as a source of constant inspiration.

Notes

1. A laryngoscope is a handheld instrument with a built-in light that is used to retract the tongue and allow the epiglottis and larynx to be viewed. The device has a protruding metal arm that is placed at the base of the tongue, enabling the tongue to be pulled up and out of the way, providing an unobstructed view of the larynx. The laryngoscope enables the placement of an endotracheal tube, a plastic tube that is inserted in between the vocal cords. One end of the tube is advanced into the lungs, the other is connected to a source of oxygen so that the lungs of unconscious patients can be ventilated. Deeply unconscious patients may not be able to breathe without an endotracheal tube because the vocal cords can close and the tongue can fall back to impede the entry of air into the lungs. The endotracheal tube prevents this problem, providing a steady flow of unimpeded air into the lungs.

2. Resuscitation is defined as the process of restoring consciousness, vigor, or life. In the setting of emergency and intensive care, when the patient is still breathing, resuscitation refers chiefly to the infusion of intravenous fluids to prevent severe dehydration. If breathing or heartbeat ceases, then cardiopulmonary resuscitation, or CPR, is performed.

3. Robert S. Gottfried, The Black Death (New York: Free Press, 1985), 45.

4. Ralph H. Major, Classic Descriptions of Disease (Springfield, Ill.: Charles C. Thomas, 1978), 77–79. Apostem is an old word meaning "abscess." Carbuncle is another word for "boil," a painful swelling of the skin caused by bacterial infection.

5. Ibid., pp. 84–85.

6. Septic shock, caused by infection, is just one type of shock.

Other types include hemorrhagic shock, caused by blood loss; cardiogenic shock, caused by heart dysfunction; and neurogenic shock, caused by inappropriate dilation of resistance arteries.

7. "Colectomy" is surgery to remove a part of the colon—usually, as in this case, to treat cancer.

8. Bacteria are identified in blood and tissue samples by incubating the samples under various conditions that cause bacteria to grow into colonies that become visible in culture dishes and flasks. Once grown in culture like this, the colonies can be studied further, and specific causative bacteria can be identified using stains, antibody markers, and other tests.

9. Meningitis is a disease caused by the infection and resulting inflammation of the tissues covering the brain and spinal cord, the meninges. Microbial causes of meningitis can be bacterial, fungal, or viral. Meningococcal meningitis is a particularly virulent and highly lethal form of meningitis caused by infection with the bacteria *Neisseria meningitidis*. These bacteria can be spread by close or prolonged contact with a patient, so people in the same household, classroom, or day-care center are at increased risk of developing the disease. Large epidemics no longer occur in the United States, but overseas travelers should check to see whether vaccination is recommended before their trip.

10. This refers to 200 cubic centimeters (cc) per kilogram (kg) of Laura's body weight. This is an enormous amount of fluid. By comparison, a typical hourly fluid rate is between one-half and one cc/kg.

11. A French catheter is a 0.079-inch-diameter plastic tube, usually used to drain the urinary bladder or some other body cavity. It is significantly wider than a standard 18-gauge intravenous catheter, which is 0.0556 inches in diameter. In this case the team inserted the large "6 French" catheter into a vein to enable the infusion of very large amounts of fluid needed to prevent death.

12. "Preload" is a measure of how much tension is on the heart as it begins to pump blood. It is measured by placing a pressure transducer into the ventricle or pulmonary artery. Drugs and fluid are used to establish optimal level of preload, in order to produce the most effective contractions of the heart. Epinephrine, or "adrenaline," is a powerful drug that increases the force of cardiac contrac-

tions and causes the blood vessels to constrict, both of which raise blood pressure.

13. The normal range for heart rate is 72 to 85 beats per minute. The normal range for blood pressure is 120–140/70–90.

14. Merriam-Webster (2004) online dictionary (www.m-w.com).

15. *The American Heritage Dictionary of the English Language*, 4th ed., as cited at Dictionary.com.

16. *Hypoxemia* is defined as abnormally low levels of oxygen in the blood. Oliguria is abnormally low urine production. Lactic acidosis is a state of acidic blood caused by the accumulation of lactic acid.

17. Richard S. Hotchkiss et al., "Apoptotic cell death in patients with sepsis, shock, and multiple organ dysfunction." *Critical Care Medicine* 27, no. 7 (July 1999): 1230–1251.

18. A collapsed lung, or "pneumothorax," can occur when air escapes from the lungs and becomes trapped between the outside of the lung and the inside of the chest wall. The resulting air pocket collapses the adjacent lung, which can no longer ventilate. A pneumothorax can be caused during a cardiac arrest, especially in small children, by overly aggressive ventilation, which can rupture the outer layer of the lung, leading to lung collapse and diminished ability to exchange oxygen and carbon dioxide.

19. C. G. Jung, *Memories, Dreams, Reflections* (New York: Vintage Books, 1989), 115–117.

20. All experiments involving animals described here and in the rest of the book, many of which led directly to the development of drugs for human patients, were overseen by an Institutional Animal Care and Use Committee, which ascertained that animals received humane and proper treatment.

21. A "paradigm" is defined as a theoretical framework that can explain a series of experimental observations and results. In his 1962 book *The Structure of Scientific Revolutions*, Thomas S. Kuhn defined the concept of a "paradigm shift" as an "intellectually violent revolution" in scientific thought. The result of a paradigm shift is that "one conceptual world view is replaced by another." The germ theory of disease is an example of a paradigm shift.

22. This quote was obtained from an interview with Professor Feldmann by William Paul. The entire transcript of the interview

can be found at http://www.laskerfoundation.org/awards/library/ 2003feldmann_int.shtml.

23. The High Mobility Group Box (HMGB) protein family members include HMGB1, HMGB2, and HMGB3. They were previously known as HMG1, HMG2, and HMG4. HMGB1 is also sometimes called "amphoterin."

24. R. A. Good, "Foreword: Interactions of the Body's Major Networks," in *Psychoneuroimmunology*, ed. R. Ader (Orlando, Fla.: Academic Press, 1981), xvii–xix.

25. J.E. Blalock, "Harnessing a Neural-immune Circuit to Control Inflammation and Shock." *Journal of Experimental Medicine* 195, no. 6 (March 18, 2002): F25–F28.

26. The complete formal name of this receptor is "alpha-7 nicotinic acetylcholine receptor subunit."

27. *Autonomic dysregulation* is abnormal function in the sympathetic and parasympathetic nervous systems.

28. See note 25.

Index

Burn unit (continued)
personnel. See Medical professionals/medical team
See also Intensive care
Burns
calculating body surface percentage of, 17–18
defined, 13
degrees and depths of wound, 16
See also Wounds

Cachectin, 130
See also Tumor necrosis factor (TNF)
Cachexia, 130
Cadavers, 62–63
donor skin, 58, 62, 63, 64
Calcium, 120
Cancer, severe sepsis development, 3
Capillaries, skin grafts and, 64
Carbolic acid, Listerization and, 142
Carbon dioxide monitoring, 52, 54
Carbuncle, 74, 207
Cardiac arrest, pediatric, 119–124
Cardiac arrhythmia, elevated potassium levels and, 94
Cardiogenic shock, 208
Cardiopulmonary resuscitation (CPR), 207
pediatric, 119, 120
Cardiovascular disease, mortality rates, 90
Catheters
bacteria at insertion point, 36, 190
femoral artery and vein catheterization, 35, 36
French, 80, 208
insertion and use of, 35–36
intra-arterial, 35–36, 52
intravenous, 9, 27, 35
needle insertion point, 36
size considerations, 27, 36
Cause of death
burn injury, 91
cardiopulmonary arrest, 126–127
on death certificates, 109
in-depth autopsy study of severe sepsis, 111–113
Cell death
apoptotic cell death, 209

cytokines and, 25
severe sepsis, 111–112
Cellular immunity, Mechnikov and, 144–145
Centocor Inc., 148
Cerami, Anthony, 129–130, 139
Cerebral function, altered, 91, 191
See also Brain function; Mental status
Cerebral ischemia, 172
Children
brain function tests, 39
burn prevention measures, 12–13
family access to, 105
injection and catheter placement for, 36
juvenile rheumatoid arthritis, 149
mortality rates and exposure to parents in hospital, 106
pediatric cardiac arrest, 119–124
results of blood volume depletion in, 61
risk and incidence of severe scald injury, 12
Cholinergic agents, excessive inflammation and, 197
Cholinergic anti-inflammatory pathway, 186–193, 199–202
desensitization (tachyphylaxis), 192–193
Chorine, 176
Chronic care, 108–109
Clinical findings, documenting, 17, 26
See also Vital signs and data
Clinical trials
anti-TNF, 150–155, 156
future, 156–157
HMGB₁, 168
CNI-₁₄₉₃ molecule, 171–174, 177, 183
Codeine, pain management, 9
Colectomy, 78, 208
Collagen, 15
skin grafts and, 64
Computed tomography (CT) scanning, 195
Controlled breathing exercises, vagus nerve and, 198–199
Core body temperature, 51
Cortisol, 42
Crohn's disease, 149

Endotracheal tube, 10, 84, 87, 94, 114, 120
  intolerability of, 86
  laryngoscope and, 207
  use during surgery, 54–55, 65
Enterobacteriaceae, 96
Epidermis, 14
Epilepsy, 187, 196
Epinephrine, 42, 80, 84, 120, 201, 208
Epithelial cells, 112–113, 114, 133
Epithelial leakage, 113, 114, 164–165
Epithelial organs, damage and failure, 112–113, 133, 164–165
Eschar
  about, 18
  bacteria in, 18–19
  bathing and debridement, 47, 58
  removal and skin replacement. See Skin grafts; Surgery
Escherichia coli, 96
Ethyl pyruvate, 163
Europe, plague, 71–76
Excessive scar formation, 117–118
Exercise, 199
Extracellular matrix of dermis, 15

Families
  access to pediatric patients, 105
  bond to medical team, 30–31
  burn unit and, 30
  comfort and hope for, 92, 104
  dialogues with, 68–70, 106–107
  emotions, 47–48
  grief and anguish at loss of loved one, 122–123
  interaction with patient, 89
  memories, 33, 203–204
  mental survival/adaptive response, 124, 125–126
  monotony of severe sepsis, 103–104
  pictures, 44–45
  postoperative reporting and dialogue with, 68–70
  progress and recovery and, 32
  support systems, 117–118
  vigilance, 104–106
Feeding and nutrition, 39–40, 42–44, 45
  See also Metabolism and metabolic rate

Feldmann, Marc, 148–149, 209
Femoral artery and vein catheterization, 35, 36
Fever, 25, 38, 93, 191
"Fight or flight" response, 42
Fink, Mitchell, 112, 163
  acute septic shock example, 78–79
First-degree burns, 16
Fleas, 143
  Yersinia pestis and, 75
Foley catheter, 37
Fong, Yuman, 139
Formalin, 63
Full-thickness burns, 16, 26

Gallbladder, 95
Germ theory of disease, 141–147
Germs. See Bacteria; Immune response; Infection
Giroir, Brett
  acute septic shock case example, 79–80
  pediatric cardiac arrest memories, 123–124
Glucocorticoids, 201
Glucose levels, 38, 52, 78, 132, 195
Good, Robert A., 176
Groin area, catheter insertion point, 35, 36

Hair follicles, 14, 15
Halothane, 55, 64
Heart, "preload," 80, 208
Heart attack, 77
Heart rate
  burn patients, 9, 37, 52
  normal, 209
  vagus nerve and, 179–181
Heartbeats, vagus nerve and, 191, 198–199
Hemorrhage, skin grafts and, 62
Hemorrhagic shock, 208
  HMGB$_1$ release and, 165
Hepatocytes, 95
Hesse, David, 139
High mobility group B$_1$ (HMGB$_1$), 22, 158–159
  acetylcholine and suppression of, 188–189
  animal studies, 160–169

shock and, 76–77, 84–85, 132, 140
slowing coagulation at sites, 195
Organ function/dysfunction, 69, 91, 115
Organs, vagus nerve system and, 183
Oxygen delivery. *See* Respirators and ventilators
Oxygen level/saturation, 52–54, 94

Pacemakers
brain and vagus nerve function manipulation, 196
cardiac, 121–122
Pain
sensation of, 15–16
of severe sepsis, 100
stimulated by immune response, 24
Pain management, 9, 27, 36, 37
Paradigm and paradigm shift, 143, 209
Parasympathetic nervous system, autonomic dysregulation, 210
Partial-thickness burns, 16, 25–26
Pasteur, Louis, 141–142, 144
Pathogens, omnipresence of, 19
Pathologists, clues about severe sepsis from, 109–112
See also Autopsy results
Patients. *See* Burn patients
Paul, William, 209
Payson 7 Burn Unit, 28–29, 44
Pediatric patients. *See* Children
Peripheral alpha-$_7$ macrophage receptor, pharmacological agents targeting, 197
Peritonitis, 157–158, 162
the Pestilence. *See* Plague
Pharmaceutical companies, monoclonal antibodies development, 147, 149
Pharmacological agents
targeting peripheral alpha-$_7$ macrophage receptor, 197
vagus nerve stimulators, 196
See also specific agents
Physical therapy and rehabilitation, 118
Physicians, bubonic syndrome and black death and, 72–73, 74
Pituitary gland, 174, 202
Plague

bubonic and septicemic, 71–76, 92, 140, 141, 156
severe sepsis comparison/contrast to, 96
transmission vector eradication, 143
Platelet count, fall in, 38, 78
Pneumonia, severe sepsis development, 3
Pneumothorax, 209
"Positive affect," 199
Post-traumatic stress disorder, 126
Postburn care, 117–118
Postoperative account
facing the realities, 68–70
next course of treatment, 69
nursing and postoperative care, 67
recovery. *See* Progress and recovery, postoperative
reporting to and dialog with family, 68–70
sensitivities and behaviors following surgery, 65–67
Potassium levels, elevated, 93–94
Prayer, 89, 114, 199
Pressure, sensation of, 15
Prieto, Dee, 160
Proceedings of the National Academy of Sciences, HMGB$_1$ study results, 163 164
Prognosis, 26
Progress and recovery, postoperative
from acute septic shock episode, 87, 154
from intensive care, 32
post-operative account, 64–65, 68
See also Treatment of burns
Proteins
Bloom's study, 158–159
metabolism of dying and, 43
as molecular weapon, 22
See also Cytokines; Tumor necrosis factor (TNF); High mobility group B$_1$ (HMGB$_1$)
Pseudomonas, 96
Psychoactive vagus nerve stimulators, 196
Public awareness of severe sepsis, 90–91
Public health and sanitation, 142–143

Tumor necrosis factor (*continued*)
shock-inducing studies in mice,
130–133, 134, 135
sudden release, 131–133
vagus nerve and, 184–186, 198–199
Tumor necrosis factor (TNF) synthesis, inhibiting, 173–174
Turnbull, Hal, 119–122

Ulcerative colitis, example, 197
Ulloa, Luis, 163, 188–189
Urinary bladder, Foley catheter and, 37
Urine output, 37, 93

Vaccines and vaccination, 144
Vagus nerve
about, 175
anti-inflammatory output, 202
behavioral conditioning and learned association and, 199–200
depressed activity and autonomic dysfunction, 191–192, 200
drug and device therapies to manipulate, 186, 196–197, 203
heart and, 198–199
heart rate regulation, 179–181
immune system regulation, 175, 181, 183–192
ligation (vagotomy), 178–179, 186–187
organs and, 183
pacemakers for, 196
stimulation and epilepsy, 187
stimulation and TNF suppression, 186–187
transmitting inflammation information, 179
Vital signs and data, 8–9
flow sheets, 38

monitoring and recording, 37–38, 44
during surgery, 51–54

Wang, Haichao, 160–161
Water, boiling, time required to cause third-degree burn, 16
Watkins, Linda, 178–179
Weight gain and weight loss, 40–41
West African meningococcal epidemic, 140
White blood cells, 64
clotting in blood vessels, 78, 132–133
count, 38, 77–78
dendritic cells, 20, 182
lymphocytes, 20, 22, 23
macrophages, 20–22, 23
mast cells, 20, 182
Mechnikov and cellular immunity, 144–145
monocytes, 20
neutrophils, 20, 22, 23, 164
polymorphonuclear leukocytes, 24
TNF and, 132–133
See also Cytokines
Wounds
appearance, 57
bathing and debridement, 47, 58
cleansing and dressing, 2, 45, 47
exposure to bacteria, 2
HMGB, release and, 165
odor, 57

Yang, Huan, 162–163
Yersin, Alexandre-Emile-John, 75
Yersinia pestis, 75–76

Other Dana Press Books and Periodicals

Books for General Readers
(available in bookstores)

THE ETHICAL BRAIN

Michael S. Gazzaniga, Ph.D.

Explores how the lessons of neuroscience can help us resolve today's ethical dilemmas, ranging from when life begins to "off-label" use of drugs such as Ritalin by students preparing for exams, and from free will and personal responsibility to public policy and religious belief. The author, a pioneer in cognitive neuroscience, is a member of the President's Council on Bioethics. 225 pp.
1-932594-01-9 $25.00

A WELL-TEMPERED MIND: Using Music to Help Children Listen and Learn

Peter Perret and Janet Fox

Five musicians enter elementary school classrooms, helping children learn about music and contributing both to higher enthusiasm and improved academic performance. This charming story gives us a taste of things to come in one of the newest areas of brain research: the effect of music on the brain. 225 pp., 12 illustrations.
1-932594-03-5 $22.95

A GOOD START IN LIFE: Understanding Your Child's Brain and Behavior from Birth to Age Six

Norbert Herschkowitz, M.D., and Elinore Chapman Herschkowitz

Updated with the latest information and new material, the authors show us how young children learn to live together in family and society and explain how brain development shapes a child's personality and behavior, discussing appropriate rule-setting, the child's moral sense, temperament, language, playing, aggression, impulse control, and empathy.
Cloth, 283 pp. 0-309-07639-0 $22.95
(Updated version with 13 illustrations) Paper, 312 pp.
0-9723830-5-0 $13.95

NEUROSCIENCE AND THE LAW: Brain, Mind, and the Scales of Justice

Brent Garland, ed.; Foreword by Mark Frankel. With commissioned papers by Michael S. Gazzaniga, Ph.D. and Megan S. Steven; Laurence Tancredi, M.D., J.D.; Henry T. Greely, J.D.; and Stephen J. Morse, J.D., Ph.D.

How discoveries in neuroscience influence criminal and civil justice, based on an invitational meeting of 26 top neuroscientists, legal scholars, attorneys, and state and federal judges convened by the Dana Foundation and the American Association for the Advancement of Science. 226 pp.
1-932594-04-3 $8.95

BEYOND THERAPY: Biotechnology and the Pursuit of Happiness.
A Report of the President's Council on Bioethics
Special Foreword by Leon R. Kass, M.D., Chairman.
Introduction by William Safire

Can biotechnology satisfy deep and familiar human desires—for better children, superior performance, ageless bodies, and happy souls? This landmark report says these possibilities present us with profound ethical challenges and choices. 376 pp.

0-1-932594-05-1 $10.95

NEUROETHICS: Mapping the Field. Conference Proceedings.
Steven J. Marcus, Editor

Proceedings of the landmark 2002 conference organized by Stanford University and the University of California, San Francisco, at which more than 150 neuroscientists, bioethics, psychiatrists and psychologists, philosophers, and professors of law and public policy debated the implications of neuroscience research findings for individual and societal decision-making. 50 illustrations. 367 pp.

0-972-3830-0-X $10.95

BACK FROM THE BRINK: How Crises Spur Doctors to New Discoveries about the Brain
Edward J. Sylvester

Goes into two academic medical centers, Columbia's New York Presbyterian and Johns Hopkins Medical Institutions, to watch a new breed of doctor, the neurointensivist, save patients with life-threatening brain injuries. 16 illustrations/photos. 296 pp.

0-9723830-4-2 $25.00

THE BARD ON THE BRAIN: Understanding the Mind Through the Art of Shakespeare and the Science of Brain Imaging
Paul Matthews, M.D., and Jeffrey McQuain, Ph.D. Foreword by Diane Ackerman

Explores the beauty and mystery of the human mind and the workings of the brain, following the path the Bard pointed out in 35 of the most famous speeches from his plays. 100 illustrations. 248 pp.

0-9723830-2-6 $35.00

STRIKING BACK AT STROKE: A Doctor-Patient Journal
Cleo Hutton, and Louis R. Caplan, M.D.

A personal account with medical guidance for anyone enduring the changes that a stroke can bring to a life, a family, and a sense of self. 15 illustrations. 240 pp.

0-9723830-1-8 $27.00

THE DANA GUIDE TO BRAIN HEALTH
Floyd E. Bloom, M.D., M. Flint Beal, M.D., and David J. Kupfer, M.D., Editors.
Foreword by William Safire

A home reference on the brain edited by three leading experts collaborating with 104 distinguished scientists and medical professionals. In easy to understand lan-

guage with cross references and advice on 72 conditions such as autism, Alzheimer's disease, multiple sclerosis, depression, and Parkinson's disease. 16 full-color pages and more than 200 black and white illustrations. 768 pp.
0-7432-0397-6 $45.00

UNDERSTANDING DEPRESSION: What We Know and
What You Can Do About It
J. Raymond DePaulo Jr., M.D., and Leslie Alan Horvitz.
Foreword by Kay Redfield Jamison, Ph.D.
What depression is, who gets it and why, what happens in the brain, troubles that come with the illness, and the treatments that work.
Cloth 304 pp. 0-471-39552-8 $24.95
Paper 296 pp. 0-471-43030-7 $14.95

KEEP YOUR BRAIN YOUNG: The Complete Guide to Physical and Emotional
Health and Longevity
Guy McKhann, M.D., and Marilyn Albert, Ph.D.
Every aspect of aging and the brain: changes in memory, nutrition, mood, sleep, and sex, as well as the later problems in alcohol use, vision, hearing, movement and balance.
Cloth 304 pp. 0-471-40792-5 $24.95
Paper 304 pp. 0-471-43028-5 $15.95

THE END OF STRESS AS WE KNOW IT
Bruce McEwen, Ph.D., with Elizabeth Norton Lasley. Foreword by Robert Sapolsky
How brain and body work under stress and how it is possible to avoid its debilitating effects.
Cloth 239 pp. 0-309-07640-4 $27.95
Paper 262 pp. 0-309-09121-7 $19.95

IN SEARCH OF THE LOST CORD: Solving the Mystery of
Spinal Cord Regeneration
Luba Vikhanski
The story of the scientists and science involved in the international scientific race to find ways to repair the damaged spinal cord and restore movement. 21 photos; 12 illustrations. 269 pp.
0-309-07437-1 $27.95

THE SECRET LIFE OF THE BRAIN
Richard Restak, M.D. Foreword by David Grubin
Companion book to the PBS series of the same name, exploring recent discoveries about the brain from infancy through old age. 201 pp.
0-309-07435-5 $35.00

THE LONGEVITY STRATEGY: How to Live to 100 Using the
Brain-Body Connection
David Mahoney and Richard Restak, M.D. Foreword by William Safire
Advice on the brain and aging well.
Cloth 250 pp. 0-471-24867-3 $22.95
Paper 272 pp. 0-471-32794-8 $14.95

STATES OF MIND: New Discoveries about How Our Brains Make Us Who We Are
Roberta Conlan, Editor
Adapted from the Dana/Smithsonian Associates lecture series by eight of the
country's top brain scientists, including the 2000 Nobel laureate in medicine, Eric
Kandel.
Cloth 214 pp. 0-471-29963-4 $24.95
Paper 224 pp. 0-471-39973-6 $18.95

Free Educational Books
(order through www.dana.org)

THE DANA SOURCEBOOK OF BRAIN SCIENCE: Resources for
Secondary and Post-Secondary Teachers and Students.

A basic introduction to brain science, its history, current understanding of the
brain, new developments, and future directions. 16 color photos; 29 black and
white photos; 26 black and white illustrations. 164 pp.

ACTS OF ACHIEVEMENT: The Role of Performing Arts Centers in Education.

Profiles of 60-plus programs, eight extended case studies, from urban and rural
communities across the United States, illustrating different approaches to performing arts-education programs in school settings. Black and white photos
throughout. 164 pp.

PLANNING AN ARTS-CENTERED SCHOOL: A Handbook

A practical guide for those interested in creating, maintaining, or upgrading arts-
centered schools. Includes curriculum and development, governance, funding,
assessment, and community participation. Black and white photos throughout.
164 pp.

Periodicals

CEREBRUM: The Dana Forum on Brain Science

A quarterly journal for general readers with feature articles, debates, and book re-
views dealing with the latest discoveries about the brain and their implications for
individuals and society.
Subscription (4 issues): $30/year ($42 foreign; $48 institutions)
To order a trial copy: call 1-877-860-0901 or write to
Cerebrum Subscriber Services
P.O. Box 573, Oxon Hill, MD 20745-0573

BRAINWORK: The Neuroscience Newsletter

A bimonthly, full-color, eight-page newsletter for general readers reporting the latest findings in brain research.
Free: order through or download from www.dana.org/books/press

BRAIN IN THE NEWS

A monthly, eight-page newspaper reprinting news and feature articles about brain research from leading newspapers and magazines in the United States and abroad during the previous month.
Free: by mail only; order through www.dana.org/books/press

IMMUNOLOGY IN THE NEWS

A quarterly, eight-page newspaper reprinting news and feature articles about immune system research, disease treatment and prevention, and biodefense from U.S. and foreign newspapers and scientific journals.
Free: by mail only; order through www.dana.org/books/press

ARTS EDUCATION IN THE NEWS

A quarterly, eight-page newspaper reprinting news and feature articles about performing arts education in the schools from leading U.S. and foreign newspapers and magazines.
Free: by mail only; order through www.dana.org/books/press

PROGRESS REPORT ON BRAIN RESEARCH

Published in March annually since 1995, the Progress Report, a publication of the Dana Alliance for Brain Initiatives, identifies the most significant findings in brain research from the previous year.
Free: order through or download from www.dana.org/books/press

BRAIN CONNECTIONS: Your Source Guide to Information on
Brain Disease and Disorders.

Pocket-size, 48-page booklet listing more than 275 organizations that help people with a brain-related disorder and those responsible for their care and treatment. A publication of the Dana Alliance for Brain Initiatives. Listings include toll-free numbers, Web site and e-mail addresses and regular mailing addresses.
Free: order through or download from www.dana.org/books/press